Barbara O'Neill's Inspired Herbal Wisdom:
Embracing Herbal Practices
and the Power of Healing

Disclaimer and/or Legal Notices

The content presented in this book is for educational and informational purposes only. While I am not a medical professional, the information compiled in this book reflects thorough research and diligent effort to present accurate interpretations of Barbara O'Neill's teachings and education. However, this book is not intended as medical advice, nor should it replace consultation with a healthcare professional.

The insights and strategies shared in this book are based on my understanding and experiences, alongside comprehensive research into Barbara O'Neill's methodologies. The recommendations and advice are intended for healthy adults. Before adopting any of the practices, remedies, or suggestions contained within this book, it is crucial to consult with your physician, particularly if you have any existing health conditions or concerns.

I have endeavored to ensure the accuracy and reliability of the information provided, but it should be noted that the field of natural health is continuously evolving. Thus, some information may become outdated or be interpreted differently as new research emerges. If any errors or inaccuracies are found within this text, I warmly welcome feedback and corrections. Please feel free to contact me via email for any suggestions or to address potential updates in future editions of this book.

This book is intended to share knowledge and inspire a holistic approach to health and wellness. However, the author does not assume responsibility for any consequences, real or perceived, from applying the information herein. Your support and constructive feedback on our page are highly appreciated, whether it be positive reinforcement or critical insights. Your input is invaluable in our mission to provide valuable and accurate content to all readers interested in natural healing and Barbara O'Neill's teachings.

A Better You Everyday Publications
email address abetteryoueveryday2022@gmail.com

www.abetteryoueveryday.com

Barbara O'Neill's Inspired Herbal Wisdom: Embracing Herbal Practices and the Power of Healing

Nature Herbal Remedies and Nature's Healing for Mind, Body, and Spirit Applications and Remedies in the O'Neill Tradition

By Margaret Willowbrook

USA
2024

TABLE OF CONTENTS

GLIMPSE INTO THE CHAPTERS AHEAD.

Chapter 1: Herbal Remedies for Respiratory Health.

In this opening chapter, we delve into the world of natural solutions for respiratory ailments. The common cold, an unwelcome yet frequent visitor, is addressed with a range of herbal remedies designed to soothe symptoms and accelerate recovery. Sore throats and coughs, often persistent and discomforting, are met with gentle yet effective herbal concoctions. For those battling sinusitis and allergies, this chapter offers a beacon of relief through natural, anti-inflammatory, and decongestant herbs. Each remedy is presented with detailed preparation instructions and tips for use, making them accessible to all.

Chapter 2: Digestive Wellness with Herbs.

The journey continues with a focus on digestive health. Here, we explore natural treatments for common digestive issues such as acid reflux, indigestion, constipation, and diarrhea. The chapter emphasizes the importance of gut health and provides a variety of herbal solutions to restore balance and comfort. Bloating and digestive discomfort, often overlooked yet crucial aspects of wellbeing, are addressed with recipes that are both palliative and preventive.

Chapter 3: Heart and Circulatory Health.

Turning our attention to the heart and circulatory system, this chapter introduces herbal remedies for managing blood pressure and cholesterol; two significant concerns in modern health. The chapter is not only about treatment but also prevention, offering insights into how certain herbs can support circulatory health, thus providing a comprehensive approach to cardiovascular wellness.

Chapter 4: Skin Care and Dermatological Health.

Skin, our largest organ, reflects our overall health and requires special attention. This chapter presents natural treatments for skin conditions such as acne, eczema, psoriasis, and rashes. Beyond treatment, it also covers herbal skincare routines that nourish and protect the skin, ensuring its health and vitality.

Chapter 5: Joint and Muscle Health.

As we progress, the focus shifts to joint and muscle health. This chapter offers a wealth of knowledge for those suffering from arthritis, joint pain, muscle aches, and strains. The healing properties of herbs come to the forefront, providing relief and improved mobility. Soothing herbal baths, a highlight of this chapter, offer both physical relief and mental relaxation.

Chapter 6: Mental and Emotional Well-being.

The connection between mind and body is undeniable, and this chapter addresses it through herbal remedies for stress, anxiety, depression, and mood swings. Sleep, a critical component of health, is also covered, with natural sleep aids and relaxation techniques that encourage restful and rejuvenating sleep.

Chapter 7: Women's and Men's Health.

Addressing the unique health needs of women and men, this chapter provides herbal solutions for hormonal balance, menstrual discomfort, menopause symptoms, and prostate health. The remedies are tailored to support the specific physiological and hormonal requirements of both genders.

Chapter 8: Herbal First Aid Kit.

Preparation is key in managing minor injuries and common ailments. This chapter serves as a guide to building an herbal first aid kit, equipped with remedies for cuts, burns, bites, headaches, migraines, and more. The focus is on quick and effective natural responses to everyday health emergencies.

Chapter 9: Seasonal Herbal Remedies.

Seasonal changes bring about specific health challenges. This chapter offers advice on adapting herbal remedies to the changing seasons. It includes immunity-boosting recipes for the cold and flu season and remedies for summer-related issues like sunburn and insect bites.

Conclusion.

In the closing section, we reflect on the journey through the world of herbal remedies and the importance of incorporating these practices for long-term health and harmony. This final note aims to inspire and encourage readers to continue exploring and integrating natural healing practices into their daily lives.

Attention!

Before you dive into this captivating book, we have an exclusive offer just for you! A fantastic FREE Bonus:

Get Your Ready-to-Print Herbal Reference Guide Bonuses!

Remedy Recipes
(6 pages)

Herbal First Aid
(4 pages)

Herb Directory
(6 pages)

EXPLORE A VARIETY OF NATURAL, EASY-TO-PREPARE REMEDY RECIPES FOR DAILY HEALTH NEEDS, SPANNING STRESS RELIEF TO IMMUNE SUPPORT.

ACCESS DETAILED HERBAL SOLUTIONS FOR COMMON HEALTH ISSUES, PROVIDING NATURAL EMERGENCY CARE ALTERNATIVES.

DELVE INTO AN EXTENSIVE DIRECTORY OF MEDICINAL HERBS, COMPLETE WITH USES, BENEFITS, AND PREPARATION TIPS.

These printable guides, crafted after extensive research and dedication, offer quick, easy access to a wealth of herbal remedies, recipes, and first aid information. Designed for fast reference, they cover everything from specific herbs in our 'Herb Directory', to swift recipes in 'Remedy Recipes', and practical emergency care in 'Herbal First Aid'. Though we plan to sell them separately in the future, we're currently offering these guides for free as our appreciation for your book purchase, as a way of saying thank you and adding extra value to your reading experience.

For instant delivery, simply chat with our Facebook bot via the link below or scan the accompanying QR code.

http://tinyurl.com/Herbalbonuses

Alternatively, you can request the guides by emailing us at: info@abetteryoueveryday.com.
Enjoy your reading and these additional resources!

INTRODUCTION OF THE BOOK.

Welcome to " Barbara O'Neill's Inspired Herbal Wisdom book" As we embark on this enlightening journey together, it is my pleasure, Margaret Willowbrook, to guide you through the gentle yet powerful world of natural remedies and holistic health. This book is more than just a guide; it's a pathway to a life enriched with the wisdom of nature, inspired by the teachings of Barbara O'Neill, a pioneer in the realm of natural health.

The core philosophy that drives this book is simple yet profound: nature holds the key to our health, well-being, and harmony. In our modern world, where technology and medicine have made remarkable strides, we often overlook the simplest solutions that nature freely offers. This book aims to bridge that gap, bringing to light the age-old wisdom of herbal remedies and natural practices that can enhance our health and enrich our lives.

The journey of compiling this book has been one of discovery, learning, and passion. Drawing from the vast pool of knowledge left behind by Barbara O'Neill, as well as from my own experiences and research, I have crafted a guide that is practical, accessible, and comprehensive. Each page is imbued with the understanding that our health is a precious gift and that taking care of it requires a holistic approach, one that considers the body, mind, and spirit as an interconnected whole.

In these pages, you will find a collection of remedies for a wide range of common ailments; from the pesky common cold to more persistent issues like digestive disorders and skin conditions. These remedies are more than just quick fixes; they are part of a larger philosophy of living in harmony with our bodies and the natural world. They are designed to not only alleviate symptoms but also to nurture and strengthen the body, promoting long-term health and vitality.

But this book is not just about treating ailments. It's also about prevention. It's about understanding how to live in a way that naturally fosters health and well-being. You will learn how the food we eat, the herbs we use, and even the way we breathe and move, all contribute to our overall health. The remedies and practices recommended in this book are complemented by advice on diet, exercise, and mindfulness, providing a holistic approach to health.

One of the fundamental principles of this book is simplicity. In a world where we are often overwhelmed by complex solutions and constant information, there is immense value in returning to the basics. The remedies presented here are simple to prepare, using ingredients that are easily accessible and often already a part of your kitchen or garden. This simplicity, however, does not compromise their effectiveness. Nature's ingredients, when used correctly, are powerful and can bring about profound changes in our health.

As we delve into the remedies and practices, you will notice that each one is more than just a list of ingredients or steps. They are presented with an understanding of why they work, how they affect the body, and when they are best used. This knowledge is crucial, as it empowers you to make informed decisions about your health and to understand the rationale behind each treatment.

Sustainability and respect for the environment are also key themes in this book. In our pursuit of health, it is important to remember that we are part of a larger ecosystem. The way we treat our bodies and the choices we make about our health have a ripple effect on the world around us. The practices and remedies in this book are in harmony with this principle, promoting health in a way that is respectful and sustainable for the environment.

In addition to physical health, this book also touches upon the importance of mental and emotional well-being. The mind and body are deeply connected, and true health encompasses both. You will find remedies and practices aimed at reducing stress, improving sleep, and enhancing overall mental and emotional balance. These practices are particularly relevant in our fast-paced, often stressful modern lives.

The journey through this book is also a personal one. Health is not a one-size-fits-all concept. Each person is unique, with their own set of needs, challenges, and circumstances. The remedies and advice in this book are meant to be adaptable, allowing you to tailor them to your personal situation. I encourage you to listen to your body, to experiment with the remedies, and to find what works best for you.

As you turn these pages, I invite you to do so with an open mind and heart. Let this book be a starting point for a deeper exploration into the world of natural health. Let it inspire you to learn more, to experiment, and to take an active role in your health journey. Remember, the path to wellness is a journey, not a destination. It is a continuous process of learning, growing, and adapting.

In conclusion, This book is more than just a compilation of remedies; it is a guide to a way of life. It is an invitation to reconnect with the wisdom of nature, to take control of your health, and to live a life of balance, health, and harmony. Join me on this journey, and let us explore the wonders of nature's pharmacy together.

FOREWORD.

In the ever-expanding world of health and wellness, where the modern complexities often overshadow the simplicity of nature, this book emerges as a guiding light. This book, deeply inspired by the teachings of Barbara O'Neill, a venerated figure in the realm of natural health, seeks to offer more than just remedies. It is an invitation to embrace a lifestyle that harmonizes with the natural rhythms of life and the wisdom inherent in the world around us.

As your author, Margaret Willowbrook, I am delighted to share this journey with you. My path has been one of continuous learning and discovery in the field of natural healing, guided by the profound insights of experts like Barbara O'Neill. Her holistic approach to health, emphasizing the balance and connection between the body, mind, and spirit, has profoundly influenced my work and this book.

Embarking on this journey, it is essential to recognize the immense value and power of the natural world in healing and maintaining our health. In every leaf, root, and flower, there is a story of healing waiting to be told. This book aims to narrate these stories in a manner that resonates with your everyday life, providing practical solutions that are both effective and harmonious with nature.

This book is not merely a collection of herbal recipes; it is a comprehensive guide designed to introduce you to a holistic way of living. It is a response to the growing need for a natural approach to health that is accessible, sustainable, and in tune with our bodies' inherent wisdom. Each chapter, each remedy,

9

is carefully crafted to bring you closer to the natural world and its abundant healing properties.

The remedies and practices outlined in this book are drawn from the rich tapestry of herbal medicine, a tradition that dates back centuries and spans across cultures and continents. These remedies have been time-tested, passed down through generations, and are rooted in a deep understanding of the natural world. They are simple, yet powerful; gentle, yet effective.

As we progress through this book, you will find that each remedy is more than a solution to a health issue; it is a step toward a life of balance and harmony. The practices recommended here are designed to align you with the rhythms of nature, to bring a sense of peace and well-being that extends beyond physical health. Whether you are new to herbal medicine or a seasoned practitioner, there is something in this book for everyone.

In writing this book, my goal has been to make herbal medicine and natural healing practices accessible to all. The remedies are simple to prepare, using ingredients that are readily available, often already part of your daily life. Each chapter is a step toward empowering you with the knowledge and skills to take charge of your health in the most natural way possible.

I encourage you to approach this book with an open mind and heart. The path to wellness is as much about healing the body as it is about nurturing the soul. Embrace the simplicity and effectiveness of these remedies, and allow them to guide you toward a healthier, more balanced existence.

This book also reflects a commitment to sustainability and ethical practices. In today's world, where the environment faces unprecedented challenges, it is more important than ever to adopt practices that are not only good for us but also for the planet. The herbal remedies and practices outlined in this book are in harmony with these principles, promoting a lifestyle that respects and protects our natural environment.

As we embark on this journey together, remember that the path to wellness is a personal one. Each of us has a unique body, mind, and set of circumstances. The remedies in this book are meant to be a starting point, a foundation upon which you can build your personal journey toward health and harmony.

In conclusion, this book is more than just a book; it is a companion on your journey to a healthier, more harmonious life. It is a tribute to the healing power of nature and a call to return to a way of life that respects and utilizes this power for our well-being. Join me in this journey of discovery, healing, and harmony, as we explore the secrets of nature's pharmacy, one remedy at a time.

Important information! Why Our Book Does Not Include colored Herb Photos!

Consideration for Cost and Accessibility:

In our commitment to keeping the book affordable, we consciously decided against including color herb photos. This decision directly impacts and lowers the printing costs, making the book more accessible to a broader range of readers. Our priority is to provide comprehensive herbal knowledge at a reasonable price.

Emphasizing the Role of Visual Aids:

Understanding the importance of visual identification in herbal studies, especially for newcomers and in recipe preparation, we recommend for detailed herb images.

https://myplantin.com/plant-identifier/herb

This online resource complements our book perfectly, enabling accurate herb identification and enhancing your herbal learning experience.

INTRODUCTION.

Welcome, this book is not just a collection of remedies and practices; it is a manifestation of a profound journey into the heart of natural healing and wellness. Inspired by the teachings of Barbara O'Neill, an esteemed figure in natural health, this book aims to bring her holistic approach to a wider audience, interpreted through my own experiences and understanding as Margaret Willowbrook.

Barbara O'Neill's philosophy on health and wellness is deeply rooted in the understanding that our bodies are incredible systems capable of self-healing and balance. She believes in the power of natural foods, herbs, and lifestyle choices to not only cure illnesses but also to prevent them. Her approach is holistic, considering the physical, emotional, and spiritual aspects of health. This philosophy resonates deeply with my own beliefs and practices, and it forms the foundation upon which this book is built.

Throughout this book, you'll discover how O'Neill's principles can be applied in practical ways to improve your daily health and well-being. Her teachings emphasize the importance of understanding the body's natural rhythms and working with them through diet, herbal remedies, and mindful practices. This approach to health is not about quick fixes or suppressing symptoms, but about nurturing the body and mind to achieve lasting wellness.

My journey into the world of natural health began years ago, fueled by a desire to find more holistic and effective ways to address health issues. Like many, I found myself disillusioned with the limitations and side effects of conventional medicine. This led me to explore alternative approaches, where I discovered the teachings of Barbara O'Neill. Her holistic view of health, which encompasses a balanced diet, the use of natural remedies, and a mindful approach to living, was a revelation. It shifted my understanding of health from being merely the absence of disease to a state of complete physical, mental, and social well-being.

In writing this book, my aim is to share the wisdom I've gleaned from years of study and practice, combined with the invaluable teachings of Barbara O'Neill. Each chapter is carefully crafted to provide practical advice and insights into using natural remedies and adopting lifestyle changes that promote health. The book covers a wide range of topics, from managing common ailments with herbal remedies to making dietary changes that support overall health.

One of the key aspects of O'Neill's philosophy is the emphasis on education and empowerment. She believes that understanding how our bodies work and the impact of our lifestyle choices on our health is crucial. This knowledge empowers us to make informed decisions and take an active role in maintaining our health. Throughout this book, you will find detailed explanations of how various remedies work, the benefits of different herbs and foods, and the science behind certain lifestyle practices. This information is presented in a way that is accessible and practical, allowing you to easily incorporate these practices into your daily life.

Another important aspect of this book is its focus on prevention. In line with O'Neill's teachings, the book emphasizes the importance of adopting a lifestyle that supports long-term health. This includes dietary advice, recommendations for physical activity, and stress management techniques. The goal is to provide you with the tools and knowledge to maintain a state of health that prevents illness from taking hold in the first place.

The book also addresses the spiritual and emotional aspects of health, which are often overlooked in conventional medicine. O'Neill's teachings recognize the interconnectedness of the mind, body, and spirit. Stress, emotions, and mental state can have a profound impact on physical health, and vice versa. This book offers guidance on practices that nurture the mind and spirit, such as meditation, mindfulness, and connecting with nature. These practices are integral to achieving a state of harmony and balance, which is the essence of true health.

In addition to focusing on individual health, this book also considers the broader context of our health choices. Sustainability and respect for the environment are integral to O'Neill's philosophy. The remedies and practices recommended in this book are not only beneficial for our health but are also mindful of their impact on the planet. This approach aligns with a growing awareness of the need to live in a way that is sustainable and harmonious with the natural world.

In conclusion, this book is a comprehensive guide to natural health and wellness. It is a blend of Barbara O'Neill's holistic health teachings and my own insights and experiences in the field of natural medicine. This book is an invitation to embark on a journey of health and wellness that is enriching, sustainable, and grounded in the wisdom of nature. It is my hope that through this book, you will find the inspiration and tools to live a healthier, more balanced, and harmonious life.

INTRODUCTION TO BARBARA O'NEILL'S PHILOSOPHY.

In the realm of natural health and wellness, Barbara O'Neill stands as a significant figure whose teachings have illuminated the path for many seeking a holistic approach to wellbeing. This subchapter aims to provide an in-depth understanding of O'Neill's philosophy, a cornerstone that shapes the content of this book.

Barbara O'Neill's approach to health is rooted deeply in the belief that the human body, given the right conditions and care, has an inherent ability to heal and maintain itself. This perspective is a departure from conventional views of medicine, where the focus is often on treating symptoms rather than addressing underlying causes. O'Neill advocates for a holistic view, considering not just the physical aspects of health but also the emotional, mental, and spiritual dimensions.

At the heart of O'Neill's philosophy is the concept of balance. Health, in her view, is a state of equilibrium where various aspects of our being; physical, emotional, mental, and spiritual, are in harmony. This balance is not static but a dynamic state that requires continuous nurturing and adjustment. O'Neill's teachings encourage individuals to become active participants in their health, understanding their bodies, and making choices that support this balance.

Nutrition plays a pivotal role in O'Neill's philosophy. She emphasizes the importance of a diet rich in natural, whole foods, which provide the body with essential nutrients to function optimally. O'Neill is a proponent of using food as medicine, a concept that dates back to ancient times but has gained renewed interest in recent years. Her dietary recommendations focus on foods that are as close to their natural state as possible; unprocessed, unrefined, and free from artificial additives.

The use of herbal remedies is another key aspect of O'Neill's approach. She views herbs not just as means of treating illness but as tools to support overall health and prevent disease. O'Neill's teachings include a deep understanding of the healing properties of various herbs and how they can be used to support different aspects of health. Her approach to herbal medicine is both practical and intuitive, encouraging individuals to learn about herbs and incorporate them into their daily lives.

Physical activity and exercise are also integral to O'Neill's holistic approach to health. She advocates for regular, moderate exercise as a way to maintain physical fitness, reduce stress, and support overall wellbeing. O'Neill's recommendations are not about intense, rigorous workouts but about finding enjoyable and sustainable ways to incorporate movement into daily life.

O'Neill also places significant emphasis on the mental and emotional aspects of health. She recognizes that stress, emotions, and mental states can have a profound impact on physical health. Her teachings include strategies for managing stress, such as mindfulness, meditation, and connecting with nature. These practices are not only beneficial for mental and emotional wellbeing but also have positive effects on physical health.

Spirituality is another aspect that O'Neill weaves into her philosophy. She believes that a connection to something greater than ourselves; connection to God, is crucial for complete wellbeing. This spiritual connection provides a sense of purpose, peace, and balance, which are essential for holistic health.

O'Neill's approach is not just about individual health but also about the broader context of our health choices. Sustainability and respect for the environment are integral to her philosophy. The choices we make about our health; from the foods we eat to the products we use; have an impact on the world around us. O'Neill encourages practices that are not only good for our health but also mindful of their impact on the planet.

In essence, Barbara O'Neill's philosophy is about living in a way that is natural, balanced, and harmonious. It is about understanding and respecting the body's natural rhythms and processes. Her teachings inspire individuals to take control of their health, to make informed choices, and to live in a way that is in harmony with the natural world.

This subchapter lays the foundation for the rest of the book, providing a comprehensive understanding of O'Neill's holistic approach to health. Her philosophy is a thread that runs through each chapter, informing the practices and remedies that are presented. As we move forward, keep in mind this holistic view, which is the essence of true health and wellbeing.

Margaret Willowbrook's Approach.

In this subchapter, we explore my personal journey, Margaret Willowbrook, into the world of natural healing and how the teachings of Barbara O'Neill have shaped my approach to health and wellness. This narrative is not just about the accumulation of knowledge and skills in herbal medicine and natural therapies; it is also a story of transformation and a testament to the power of holistic healing.

My journey began in the serene countryside of the UK, where the natural world was an integral part of everyday life. From a young age, I was fascinated by the plants and herbs that grew around me, instinctively sensing their significance beyond mere landscape beautification. This early connection with nature laid the foundation for what would become a lifelong pursuit of understanding and harnessing the healing powers of the natural world.

As I grew older, my interest in natural health evolved into a more formal quest for knowledge. I was drawn to the teachings of renowned natural health practitioners, among whom Barbara O'Neill was a prominent figure. Her holistic approach to health; viewing the body as an interconnected system and emphasizing the importance of treating the whole person; resonated deeply with me. It was a stark contrast to the conventional medical practices that often focus narrowly on symptoms and diseases.

Adopting O'Neill's teachings, I began to view health not just as the absence of illness but as a state of complete physical, mental, and emotional well-being. This perspective shifted my approach from one of merely treating ailments to one of nurturing overall health and preventing disease. I started to explore various natural therapies, including herbal medicine, nutrition, and lifestyle modifications, integrating them into my own life and later, in my practice as a natural health advisor.

My approach, much like O'Neill's, is grounded in the belief that our bodies have an innate ability to heal themselves, given the right support. This support comes in many forms; through the foods we eat, the herbs we use, the air we breathe, and even the thoughts we entertain. Every aspect of our lives contributes to our overall health, and it is by addressing these various aspects that we can achieve true wellness.

In this book, my approach to natural health is presented in a way that is practical and accessible. The remedies and practices are designed to be easily integrated into daily life, regardless of one's background or experience with natural health. They are based on the principles of simplicity, effectiveness, and harmony with nature.

One of the key elements of my approach is the use of food as medicine. Nutrition plays a crucial role in maintaining health and preventing disease. The remedies and dietary advice in this book reflect this principle, emphasizing whole, unprocessed foods rich in nutrients. I believe in the healing power of food and the importance of eating in a way that supports our body's natural processes.

Herbal medicine is another cornerstone of my approach. Herbs are nature's gift to us, offering a natural way to support health and treat illness. The herbal remedies in this book are based on traditional knowledge and modern research. They are selected for their effectiveness, safety, and ease of use. I also emphasize the importance of understanding how herbs work and how to use them responsibly.

In addition to herbal remedies and nutrition, my approach also includes lifestyle practices that support overall well-being. This includes physical activity, stress management techniques, and practices that promote mental and emotional health. I believe that a balanced lifestyle is key to maintaining health and preventing illness.

My approach is also holistic in the true sense of the word. It recognizes the interconnectedness of the physical, mental, emotional, and spiritual aspects of our being. Health issues are often a manifestation of imbalances in one or more of these areas. Therefore, the remedies and practices in this book are designed to address not just physical ailments but also to promote balance and harmony in all aspects of our being.

Another important aspect of my approach is the emphasis on empowerment and education. I believe that knowledge is power, and by understanding our bodies and the principles of natural health, we can become active participants in our own healing journey. This book is designed to provide you with the knowledge and tools to take charge of your health, to make informed decisions, and to live a life that is in harmony with your body and the natural world.

Finally, my approach is grounded in respect for the environment and sustainability. I believe that our health is intimately connected to the health of the planet. The practices and remedies recommended in this book are not only beneficial for our health but also considerate of their impact on the environment. This includes using sustainable, ethically sourced ingredients and promoting practices that are in harmony with nature.

In conclusion, my approach to health and wellness, as presented in this book, is a comprehensive, holistic, and practical guide to living a healthier, more balanced life. It is an approach that is rooted in the wisdom of nature, inspired by the teachings of Barbara O'Neill, and shaped by my own experiences and understanding. It is my hope that this book will inspire you to embrace the power of natural healing and to embark on a journey toward a healthier, more harmonious life.

Chapter 1: Herbal Remedies for Respiratory Health.

In this first chapter we focus on a crucial aspect of health: the respiratory system. This chapter is dedicated to herbal remedies that have been time-honored for their efficacy in treating common respiratory ailments. The significance of respiratory health can hardly be overstated, as it is fundamental to our vitality and overall well-being.

The respiratory system, a vital gateway between our body and the environment, is often the first line of defense against airborne pathogens and pollutants. It's also frequently the first system to be affected by seasonal changes, environmental factors, and common pathogens. The ailments associated with the respiratory system, such as the common cold, sore throats, coughs, sinusitis, and allergies, while often not life-threatening, can significantly impact our quality of life and productivity.

The common cold, a ubiquitous companion especially during the colder months, is more than just an inconvenience. It is a clear signal from our body indicating the need for rest and healing. Despite the advances in modern medicine, the common cold continues to elude a cure, making symptom management and immune support essential. This is where the age-old wisdom of herbal remedies comes into play.

Herbal remedies offer a gentle yet effective means of alleviating the symptoms of the common cold. Unlike conventional treatments that often mask symptoms, these natural solutions aim to support the body's natural healing processes. Herbal teas and inhalants, for instance, have been used for centuries to provide relief from congestion, sore throats, and coughs. They work not just on the surface but at a deeper level, enhancing the body's immune response and providing a holistic healing experience.

Moving on from the common cold, we encounter other frequent irritants: sore throats and coughs. These symptoms, while often associated with colds, can arise independently due to a variety of factors including allergies, dry air, and vocal strain. A sore throat can range from a mild irritation to a severe discomfort, hindering our ability to communicate effectively and comfortably. Coughs, which serve the purpose of clearing our airways, can become troublesome if persistent.

The herbal remedies for sore throats and coughs presented in this chapter are selected for their soothing and healing properties. They not only provide immediate relief but also address underlying causes like inflammation and infection. Herbs have unique compounds that act as natural soothers and anti-inflammatories, making them ideal for these conditions.

Furthermore, the chapter addresses more chronic and often debilitating conditions like sinusitis and allergies. Sinusitis, the inflammation of the sinus passages, can be acutely painful and can significantly affect one's quality of life. Allergies, on the other hand, are a testament to the body's heightened response to certain environmental triggers. Both these conditions can be chronic and require a more strategic approach to manage.

Herbal solutions for sinusitis and allergies focus on reducing inflammation, clearing congestion, and boosting the body's natural resilience. Many herbs possess natural anti-inflammatory and decongestant properties, making them effective alternatives to over-the-counter medications. These herbs work synergistically with the body to alleviate symptoms and promote long-term respiratory health.

In this chapter, you will find an array of remedies; from simple teas and tinctures to more complex herbal blends and inhalants. Each remedy is carefully described with its preparation method and usage guidelines. These remedies are more than just a quick fix; they are part of a lifestyle that emphasizes prevention and maintenance of health.

The remedies are grounded in the understanding that each individual is unique, and what works for one may not work for another. Therefore, a variety of options are provided, allowing for personalization based on individual needs, preferences, and responses.

In summary, this chapter serves as a comprehensive guide to managing and improving respiratory health through natural means. It encourages readers to turn to nature for solutions and to understand their bodies better. It is a testament to the healing power of herbs and a tribute to the wisdom that has been passed down through generations. As we move through the chapter, readers are invited to explore these remedies, to experience the gentle yet profound healing power of nature, and to embrace a more natural approach to respiratory health.

COMMON COLD REMEDIES.

The onset of a common cold, with its all-too-familiar symptoms of a runny nose, sore throat, and sneezing, often signals a time for rest and healing. In this subchapter, we explore an array of herbal remedies designed to alleviate these symptoms and bolster the body's natural defenses. These remedies are rooted in traditional practices and are backed by a deep understanding of herbal properties.

The common cold, while not a severe illness, can be quite debilitating and uncomfortable. It's a sign from our body urging us to slow down and take care. The herbal remedies outlined here are not just about suppressing symptoms but are aimed at supporting the body's healing process and enhancing overall immunity.

One of the most effective ways to combat the onset of a cold is through herbal teas. These warm, soothing drinks do more than just provide hydration; they are packed with beneficial compounds that help fight infection and reduce symptoms. For instance, a simple ginger tea, made by slicing fresh ginger and steeping it in hot water, can work wonders. Ginger has natural anti-inflammatory and antimicrobial properties, making it an ideal remedy for colds. Adding a spoonful of honey, which has antibacterial properties, and a squeeze of lemon, rich in Vitamin C, enhances the healing properties of this tea.

Another effective remedy is the age-old echinacea tea. Echinacea is known for its immune-boosting properties and is particularly effective when taken at the onset of a cold. To prepare, steep echinacea leaves or flowers in hot water. Add a bit of honey for sweetness and its soothing effect on sore throats.

For those suffering from nasal congestion, steam inhalation with essential oils can provide immediate relief. Eucalyptus oil, with its strong, menthol-like fragrance, is particularly effective. Add a few drops of eucalyptus oil to a bowl of hot water, drape a towel over your head, and inhale the steam. This helps open up the nasal passages and has a calming effect.

Another beneficial practice is a warm bath with added herbs or essential oils. A bath infused with lavender and chamomile not only helps soothe the body but also aids in relaxation and ensures a good night's sleep, which is crucial for recovery. Lavender and chamomile have calming properties that help reduce stress, a common aggravator of cold symptoms.

Garlic, though not typically associated with tea, is a powerful natural remedy for colds. It has strong antimicrobial properties and can boost the immune system. A simple way to incorporate garlic is to finely chop a clove and mix it with honey. This mixture can be taken directly or added to tea.

For a sore throat, a sage gargle can be particularly soothing. Sage has natural antiseptic properties. To make a sage gargle, steep sage leaves in hot water, strain, and let it cool. Gargling with this solution several times a day can provide relief from sore throat pain.

Another effective remedy for cold relief is thyme tea. Thyme is known for its antispasmodic properties, making it excellent for coughs. To make thyme tea, steep dried thyme in hot water, strain, and drink. It helps in loosening mucus and eases coughing.

In addition to these remedies, it's important to maintain hydration and rest. Drinking plenty of fluids, such as water and herbal teas, helps thin mucus and keeps the throat moist, alleviating cough and sore throat symptoms. Rest is crucial as it allows the body to direct its energy towards fighting off the cold virus.

In conclusion, the remedies presented in this subchapter are practical, easy to prepare, and effective. They are rooted in a holistic approach to health, aimed at not only treating the symptoms of a common cold but also at supporting the body's overall healing process. These remedies are a testament to the power of nature in providing relief and promoting health. As with any natural remedy, it's essential to listen to your body and adjust as needed. These remedies are meant to be part of a comprehensive approach to health, one that values the wisdom of traditional practices and the healing power of nature.

SORE THROATS AND COUGHS

In this subchapter dedicated to sore throats and coughs, we delve into practical, herbal-based remedies that focus on alleviating discomfort and promoting healing. Sore throats and coughs, while often symptoms of broader conditions like colds or allergies, can be distressing and uncomfortable in their own right. The remedies provided here are crafted with care, drawing from a deep well of herbal knowledge to offer soothing relief and healing support.

Sore Throat Remedies.
A sore throat can range from a mild irritation to a severe ache, hindering speech, swallowing, and general comfort. The following remedies are designed to address various sore throat causes, from dryness and irritation to inflammation and infection.

- Licorice Root Gargle: Licorice root is a soothing herb known for its ability to ease throat pain. To prepare a licorice gargle, steep one tablespoon of dried licorice root in a cup of boiling water for about 15 minutes. Let it cool to a safe temperature and gargle with it several times a day. This not only soothes the throat but also helps reduce inflammation.

- Honey and Turmeric Paste: Honey, with its natural antibacterial properties, combined with turmeric's anti-inflammatory abilities, makes for a powerful sore throat remedy. Mix a teaspoon of turmeric powder with enough honey to form a paste. This mixture can be taken orally, slowly dissolving in the mouth, a few times a day.

- Marshmallow Root Tea: Marshmallow root contains mucilage, which coats and soothes sore throats. Boil a tablespoon of dried marshmallow root in water, strain, and drink this tea two to three times a day. Its soothing effect is almost immediate.

- Slippery Elm Lozenges: Slippery elm also contains mucilage and works similarly to marshmallow root. Slippery elm lozenges are readily available and can be used several times a day to soothe a sore throat.

Cough Remedies.
Coughs can be productive (with phlegm) or dry and are often a reflex to clear the airways. The following remedies focus on soothing the cough reflex and helping clear mucus for productive coughs.

- Thyme and Honey Syrup: Thyme has been traditionally used to treat respiratory conditions, including coughs. To make thyme syrup, simmer a handful of thyme leaves in water for 30 minutes. Strain and mix with an equal part of honey. Take a teaspoon as needed for cough relief.

- Pine Needle Tea: Pine needles are rich in vitamin C and have been used historically to treat coughs. Steep a handful of washed pine needles in boiling water for 10 minutes, strain, and drink this tea a couple of times a day. It's especially effective for dry coughs.

- Ginger and Lemon Tea: Ginger, with its anti-inflammatory properties, can help soothe a cough. Boil fresh ginger slices in water, add lemon juice, and honey to taste. This warm tea can be consumed throughout the day to provide relief from coughing.

- Onion and Honey Syrup: Onions have expectorant properties, making them effective in treating coughs. Chop an onion and cover it with honey. Let it sit for several hours, and then take a teaspoon of the syrup as needed. This remedy is particularly good for productive coughs as it helps loosen mucus.

- Peppermint Steam Inhalation: Peppermint contains menthol, which can help soothe the throat and act as a decongestant, aiding in cough relief. Boil water and add a few drops of peppermint essential oil. Inhale the steam to help alleviate coughing.

Additional Tips.
When dealing with sore throats and coughs, it's important to stay hydrated. Drinking plenty of fluids helps thin mucus and keeps the throat moist. Warm broths and herbal teas are especially beneficial. Additionally, maintaining a humid environment can prevent the drying of the throat and airways, which often exacerbates these conditions.

In summary, these remedies are crafted to provide relief from the discomfort and irritation of sore throats and coughs. They are practical and can be easily prepared with common ingredients. While these remedies are effective in providing symptomatic relief, it's important to remember that if symptoms persist or worsen, consulting a healthcare professional is advised. These remedies reflect a holistic approach to health, emphasizing natural, body-supportive treatments that work in harmony with our body's own healing processes.

SINUSITIS AND ALLERGIES.

Sinusitis and allergies are common ailments that can significantly affect the quality of life, causing discomfort and inconvenience. This subchapter is dedicated to exploring herbal solutions for these conditions, focusing on the anti-inflammatory and decongestant properties of various herbs. These natural remedies are designed to provide relief and promote healing, offering a gentler and often more harmonious alternative to conventional treatments.

Sinusitis, an inflammation of the sinuses, can lead to symptoms such as a stuffy nose, pain in the face, and even headaches. Allergies, on the other hand, can trigger reactions like sneezing, itching, and watery eyes. Both conditions can be chronic and require careful, consistent management. The herbal remedies detailed in this subchapter aim to address the root causes of these conditions, not just their symptoms.

One effective remedy for sinusitis is a steam inhalation with essential oils. Eucalyptus and peppermint oils are particularly beneficial due to their decongestant properties. To prepare this remedy, boil water and pour it into a bowl. Add a few drops of eucalyptus and peppermint essential oils. Cover your head with a towel and inhale the steam. This method helps open up the sinuses and facilitates breathing.

Nettle tea is another excellent remedy for both sinusitis and allergies. Nettle has natural antihistamine properties, making it effective in reducing allergic reactions. To make nettle tea, steep dried nettle leaves in hot water for about 10 minutes. Strain and drink this tea two to three times a day. This herbal tea can reduce inflammation and alleviate allergy symptoms.

For a more direct approach to sinus relief, a saline nasal rinse can be effective. This can be enhanced with herbs such as goldenseal, which has natural antibacterial properties. To prepare a herbal saline rinse, mix a teaspoon of salt and a pinch of goldenseal powder in warm water. Use this solution in a nasal spray bottle or a neti pot to rinse the nasal passages.

Bromelain, an enzyme found in pineapples, is known for its anti-inflammatory properties and can be particularly helpful in reducing nasal swelling in sinusitis. Bromelain supplements are available, or you can incorporate more pineapple into your diet.

Another helpful remedy for sinusitis is turmeric milk, also known as golden milk. Turmeric contains curcumin, a compound with potent anti-inflammatory properties. Warm a cup of milk (dairy or plant-based) and stir in a teaspoon of turmeric powder, a pinch of black pepper, and a sweetener of your choice. This comforting drink can help reduce sinus inflammation.

For those suffering from allergies, a tea made from butterbur can be beneficial. Butterbur is believed to block some of the chemicals that trigger allergic reactions. Steep butterbur leaves in hot water to make tea. However, it's important to use butterbur products that are certified free of pyrrolizidine alkaloids, which can be harmful to the liver.

Quercetin, a natural compound found in capers, apples, and onions, is known for its ability to stabilize mast cells and reduce the release of histamine, which causes allergy symptoms. Including these foods in your diet or taking quercetin supplements can help manage allergies.

A lesser-known remedy for allergies is stinging nettle capsules. Stinging nettle can be effective in reducing the amount of histamine the body produces in response to an allergen. It's available in capsule form, which can be a convenient way to take this herb.

In addition to these remedies, maintaining a diet low in inflammatory foods can help manage both sinusitis and allergies. Foods high in antioxidants and omega-3 fatty acids, such as berries, nuts, and fatty fish, can support the body's natural anti-inflammatory processes.

It's also beneficial to consider environmental factors that may exacerbate sinusitis and allergies. Keeping the living space free of dust, using air purifiers, and avoiding known allergens can play a significant role in managing these conditions.

In conclusion, this subchapter offers a comprehensive approach to managing sinusitis and allergies through herbal remedies. The focus is on natural, body-friendly treatments that work in harmony with our system, offering relief and promoting healing. While these remedies can be highly effective, it's important to remember that individual responses can vary. It's always advisable to consult with a healthcare professional, especially in cases of severe or persistent symptoms. These herbal solutions are part of a broader lifestyle approach that values the wisdom of natural healing and the importance of living in harmony with our bodies.

Chapter 2: Digestive Wellness with Herbs.

Welcome to the second chapter where we explore the integral role of herbs in maintaining and restoring digestive health. The digestive system is a complex and vital part of our body, playing a crucial role in overall health and wellbeing. It's not just about the food we eat but how our body processes and assimilates this food. Digestive disturbances like acid reflux, indigestion, constipation, diarrhea, and bloating can significantly impact our daily lives. This chapter aims to offer a comprehensive guide to managing these common digestive issues using herbal remedies and dietary modifications.

The holistic approach to digestive wellness recognizes that digestion is more than a physical process; it's influenced by various factors including diet, stress, lifestyle, and emotional state. A holistic approach looks at treating the underlying causes of digestive issues, not just the symptoms. It acknowledges that each individual's digestive system is unique and thus requires personalized care and treatment.

Acid reflux and indigestion are common complaints. These conditions are often a result of modern dietary habits that include processed foods, excessive caffeine, and sugar, combined with a high-stress lifestyle. Herbal remedies and dietary changes can be highly effective in alleviating these conditions. Herbs like ginger, licorice root, and chamomile have properties that soothe the digestive tract, reduce inflammation, and balance stomach acid. These herbs, used in teas or as supplements, can provide immediate relief and long-term benefits.

In addition to herbal treatments, dietary modifications play a crucial role in managing acid reflux and indigestion. This involves not only what we eat but how we eat. Mindful eating practices, such as eating slowly and chewing thoroughly, can greatly improve digestion. Incorporating foods that are high in fiber, and low in fat and sugar, can also help maintain a healthy digestive system.

Constipation and diarrhea are two sides of the same coin, representing an imbalance in the digestive process. Herbal treatments for these conditions focus on restoring this balance. For constipation, herbs like psyllium husk, senna, and aloe vera can be effective. These herbs act as natural laxatives, helping to stimulate bowel movements. However, their use should be balanced with adequate hydration and dietary fiber.

Diarrhea, on the other hand, requires a gentler approach. Herbs like slippery elm and marshmallow root can soothe the digestive tract and firm up stools. It's also important to replenish lost fluids and electrolytes with hydrating drinks.

Bloating and digestive discomfort are often a result of poor digestion, imbalanced gut flora, or food intolerances. Carminative herbs like fennel, peppermint, and caraway can be immensely helpful in reducing gas and bloating. These herbs aid in digestion, helping to break down food more efficiently and relieve discomfort.

A significant aspect of managing bloating and digestive discomfort is understanding and addressing food intolerances or sensitivities. This may involve keeping a food diary to identify triggers and making dietary adjustments accordingly.

In addressing these digestive issues, it's important to consider the interconnectedness of the body's systems. Stress management and emotional wellbeing play a significant role in digestive health. Practices such as yoga, meditation, and regular exercise can not only reduce stress but also improve digestive function.

This chapter, focusing on digestive wellness with herbs, provides practical, effective solutions for common digestive issues. It combines traditional herbal wisdom with modern understanding, offering a balanced and comprehensive approach to digestive health. The remedies and advice presented here aim to empower readers to take control of their digestive health through natural, holistic means. Remember, a healthy digestive system is a cornerstone of overall health and wellbeing. By taking care of our digestion, we nurture our entire being.

ACID REFLUX AND INDIGESTION REMEDIES.

Acid reflux and indigestion are prevalent digestive issues that many individuals experience. These conditions can cause discomfort ranging from mild heartburn to severe gastrointestinal distress. This subchapter focuses on natural remedies and dietary advice to alleviate these conditions, providing practical, herbal-based solutions.

Acid reflux, often characterized by a burning sensation in the chest or throat, occurs when stomach acid flows back into the esophagus. Indigestion, on the other hand, can manifest as bloating, gas, or an upset stomach, often after eating. While occasional occurrences are common, frequent episodes may require a more attentive approach to diet and lifestyle.

Herbal remedies have been used for centuries to treat digestive issues, and their efficacy is increasingly supported by scientific research. These natural solutions offer a gentler alternative to over-the-counter medications, addressing not only the symptoms but also the underlying causes of acid reflux and indigestion.

One effective remedy for acid reflux is a soothing tea made from marshmallow root. Marshmallow root contains mucilaginous compounds that form a protective layer in the digestive tract, reducing irritation caused by stomach acid. To prepare the tea, steep two teaspoons of dried marshmallow root in a cup of hot water for 10 minutes. Strain and drink up to three times a day, preferably between meals.

Chamomile tea is another excellent remedy for both acid reflux and indigestion. Chamomile has anti-inflammatory properties that can soothe the digestive tract and reduce stomach acid irritation. It also relaxes the muscles of the digestive tract, helping to relieve indigestion symptoms. Steep dried chamomile flowers in hot water for about 5 minutes, strain, and enjoy the tea after meals.

Slippery elm bark is a traditional remedy known for its effectiveness in treating indigestion and acid reflux. The inner bark of slippery elm contains compounds that become a slick gel when mixed with water, coating and soothing the stomach and esophagus. Mix one teaspoon of slippery elm bark powder with a cup of hot water to create a thin gruel. Consume this mixture up to three times a day.

Apple cider vinegar is a popular home remedy for indigestion, despite its acidic nature. It is believed to balance stomach acid and improve digestion. Mix one tablespoon of organic apple cider vinegar with a cup of water and drink before meals. However, this remedy may not be suitable for everyone, especially those with severe acid reflux.

Ginger is renowned for its gastrointestinal benefits, especially in relieving indigestion and nausea. Ginger tea can be made by simmering slices of fresh ginger in water for about 20 minutes. Drinking ginger tea before or after meals can help stimulate digestion and prevent indigestion.

In addition to these herbal remedies, dietary modifications can significantly impact managing acid reflux and indigestion. It is crucial to identify and avoid foods that trigger symptoms. Common triggers include spicy foods, caffeine, alcohol, and fatty foods. Eating smaller, more frequent meals rather than large meals can also help reduce the occurrence of these conditions.

Incorporating high-fiber foods into the diet is beneficial for digestive health. Fiber aids in digestion and can prevent the overproduction of stomach acid. Foods rich in fiber, such as whole grains, vegetables, and fruits, should be a staple in the diet.

Staying hydrated is essential for digestive health, but it is advisable to avoid drinking large amounts of liquids during meals, as this can dilute stomach acid and impair digestion. Instead, focus on hydrating between meals.

Maintaining a healthy weight and engaging in regular physical activity can also reduce the frequency and severity of acid reflux and indigestion. Excess weight can put pressure on the stomach, causing acid to flow back into the esophagus, while exercise aids in digestion and overall digestive health.

Stress management is another crucial aspect of treating indigestion and acid reflux. High levels of stress can exacerbate these conditions. Incorporating stress-reducing practices such as yoga, meditation, or deep breathing exercises into your daily routine can have a positive effect on digestive health.

In conclusion, this subchapter provides a comprehensive guide to treating acid reflux and indigestion using herbal remedies and dietary adjustments. These natural solutions focus on soothing the digestive system, balancing stomach acid, and improving overall digestive function. By adopting these practices, you can manage and alleviate the discomfort associated with acid reflux and indigestion, leading to improved digestive health and overall wellbeing.

Constipation and Diarrhea – Herbal Treatments.

Constipation and diarrhea are two common digestive issues that, while seemingly opposite, often stem from similar imbalances within the digestive system. This subchapter offers a deep dive into herbal treatments for both conditions, focusing on creating a balanced approach that utilizes gentle, effective herbal laxatives and astringents. These natural remedies aim to not only provide relief but also to restore normal function to the digestive system.

Constipation Remedies:

Constipation is characterized by infrequent bowel movements, difficulty passing stools, or a feeling of incomplete evacuation. It can be caused by a variety of factors including diet, lack of exercise, dehydration, and stress. Herbal remedies for constipation often focus on stimulating bowel movements and softening stools.

- Senna Tea: Senna is a potent herbal laxative known for its ability to stimulate bowel movements. It contains compounds called sennosides, which irritate the lining of the bowel, causing a laxative effect. To make senna tea, steep a senna tea bag or a teaspoon of senna leaves in hot water for 5-10 minutes. It is important to use senna sparingly as overuse can lead to dependency and dehydration.

- Psyllium Husk: Psyllium is a fiber-rich herb that absorbs water, helping to soften stools and promote regularity. Mix one to two teaspoons of psyllium husk in a glass of water and drink immediately, followed by another glass of water. It's crucial to stay well-hydrated when using psyllium husk to prevent further constipation.

- Dandelion Root Tea: Dandelion root acts as a mild laxative and helps stimulate digestion. To make the tea, simmer one teaspoon of dandelion root in a cup of water for 10 minutes. Drink this tea up to three times a day to help alleviate constipation.

- Aloe Vera Juice: Aloe vera contains compounds that have a laxative effect. Drinking aloe vera juice can help increase water content in the intestines and stimulate bowel movements. It is advisable to start with a small dose, as aloe vera can be quite potent.

- Castor Oil: Castor oil is a traditional remedy for constipation. It works as a stimulant laxative, increasing the movement of the intestines. Take one to two tablespoons of castor oil on an empty stomach. Be cautious with the dosage, as castor oil is a powerful laxative.

Diarrhea Remedies:

Diarrhea is characterized by loose, watery stools and can be caused by infections, certain medications, or digestive disorders. Herbal treatments for diarrhea aim to reduce intestinal inflammation, slow down bowel movements, and absorb excess fluid.

- Chamomile Tea: Chamomile has anti-inflammatory properties that can help soothe the digestive tract and reduce the frequency of diarrhea. Brew chamomile tea by steeping dried chamomile flowers in hot water for about 5 minutes.

- Peppermint Tea: Peppermint can relax the muscles of the digestive tract and may help relieve diarrhea. Steep dried peppermint leaves in hot water for 10 minutes, strain, and drink the tea.

- Slippery Elm Bark: Slippery elm has a high mucilage content, which can help coat and soothe the intestines, providing relief from diarrhea. Mix one teaspoon of slippery elm powder with water to create a smooth mixture and consume immediately.

- Blackberry Leaf Tea: Blackberry leaves contain tannins that can help tighten the mucous membranes in the intestines, reducing the passage of watery stools. Steep blackberry leaves in hot water for about 10 minutes, strain, and drink the tea.

- Ginger Tea: Ginger can help reduce intestinal spasms and gas associated with diarrhea. Boil slices of fresh ginger in water for 20 minutes, strain, and drink the tea. Ginger is especially effective in cases of diarrhea caused by gastroenteritis.

Dietary Considerations:

In addition to herbal remedies, dietary changes are crucial in managing both constipation and diarrhea. For constipation, a diet rich in fiber from fruits, vegetables, and whole grains is beneficial. Adequate hydration is equally important, as water helps soften stools and promotes regular bowel movements.

For diarrhea, it's advisable to follow a bland diet, including foods like bananas, rice, applesauce, and toast (BRAT diet). These foods are easy on the digestive system and can help firm up stools. It's also important to stay hydrated, as diarrhea can lead to dehydration.

In summary, this subchapter provides practical, herbal-based solutions for constipation and diarrhea, focusing on restoring balance and function to the digestive system. These remedies are complemented by dietary advice to ensure a holistic approach to treatment. While these herbal solutions can be highly effective, it's important to consult with a healthcare professional in cases of severe or persistent symptoms. Remember, the goal is not just to alleviate symptoms but to support the body's natural digestive processes and promote overall digestive wellness.

BLOATING AND DIGESTIVE DISCOMFORT – PRACTICAL SOLUTIONS.

Bloating and digestive discomfort are common issues that many people experience regularly. These symptoms can be caused by various factors, including dietary choices, stress, and digestive imbalances. This subchapter offers a comprehensive guide to managing bloating and digestive discomfort using carminative herbs and specific dietary adjustments. The remedies and tips provided here are aimed at not only alleviating symptoms but also at addressing the underlying causes of these digestive issues.

Bloating is often a result of excess gas in the digestive system or a sign of a sluggish digestive process. Digestive discomfort can manifest as a feeling of fullness, abdominal pain, or irregular bowel movements. The goal of the remedies presented here is to enhance digestion, regulate bowel movements, and reduce gas and bloating.

Herbal Remedies for Bloating and Digestive Discomfort:

- Fennel Seed Tea: Fennel seeds are excellent for relieving bloating and gas due to their carminative properties. They help relax the muscles in the digestive tract and aid in expelling gas. To make fennel tea, crush a teaspoon of fennel seeds and steep them in a cup of boiling water for 10 minutes. Strain and drink this tea after meals to aid digestion and relieve bloating.

- Peppermint Tea: Peppermint is another carminative herb that can soothe digestive discomfort. It relaxes the digestive tract muscles and can relieve symptoms of bloating and gas. Brew a cup of peppermint tea by steeping dried peppermint leaves in hot water for 5-10 minutes. This tea is particularly beneficial after meals.

- Ginger and Lemon Tea: Ginger is known for its ability to stimulate digestion and reduce inflammation in the digestive tract. Lemon, on the other hand, can help flush toxins from the digestive system. Combine slices of fresh ginger and a few slices of lemon in boiling water, steep for 10 minutes, and enjoy this soothing tea throughout the day.

- Caraway Seed Infusion: Caraway seeds have long been used to treat digestive issues, including bloating. They contain compounds that can relieve gas and improve digestion. Crush a teaspoon of caraway seeds, steep in boiling water for about 10 minutes, and drink this infusion to alleviate digestive discomfort.

- Chamomile Tea: Chamomile is not only calming but also beneficial for digestive health. It can relieve bloating and soothe gastrointestinal irritation. Brew chamomile tea by steeping dried chamomile flowers in hot water for about 5 minutes. Drinking chamomile tea in the evening can also aid in relaxation and promote better sleep.

Dietary Adjustments for Digestive Wellness:

In addition to herbal remedies, making specific dietary adjustments is crucial in managing bloating and digestive discomfort. The following tips can help enhance digestive health:

- Increase Fiber Intake: Fiber is essential for healthy digestion. It helps regulate bowel movements and prevent constipation, a common cause of bloating. Incorporate fiber-rich foods like whole grains, vegetables, fruits, and legumes into your diet.

- Stay Hydrated: Adequate hydration is key to maintaining good digestive health. It helps in the digestion of food and the absorption of nutrients. Drink plenty of water throughout the day, and consider herbal teas and infused water for variety.

- Eat Mindfully: Eating quickly or while distracted can lead to swallowing air, which contributes to bloating. Take time to eat slowly, chew your food thoroughly, and focus on the act of eating.

- Limit Intake of Gas-Producing Foods: Certain foods like beans, cabbage, and carbonated beverages can increase gas production. While it's not necessary to eliminate these foods completely, moderating their intake can help reduce bloating.

- Probiotics for Gut Health: Probiotics help balance the gut flora, which is essential for proper digestion. Include probiotic-rich foods like yogurt, kefir, sauerkraut, and kimchi in your diet, or consider a probiotic supplement.

- Avoid Artificial Sweeteners: Some artificial sweeteners can cause bloating and gas, especially in individuals with sensitivities. Be mindful of your intake of these sweeteners and consider natural alternatives.

- Regular Physical Activity: Regular exercise can enhance digestion and reduce the likelihood of constipation and bloating. Even a daily walk can significantly improve digestive health.

In conclusion, this subchapter offers a holistic approach to managing bloating and digestive discomfort. By combining herbal remedies with specific dietary adjustments, you can effectively alleviate symptoms and support overall digestive health. These natural strategies focus on enhancing digestion, regulating bowel movements, and reducing gas production. Remember, a healthy digestive system is a cornerstone of overall well-being, and taking care of it through these natural means can lead to significant improvements in health and quality of life.

CHAPTER 3: HEART AND CIRCULATORY HEALTH.

In Chapter 3 is devoted to the heart and circulatory system, which are pivotal to our overall health. The heart, a tireless muscle, and the intricate network of blood vessels work in harmony to sustain life by delivering oxygen and nutrients to every cell in the body. Maintaining the health of this system is crucial, and this chapter delves into natural approaches for managing blood pressure, cholesterol, and supporting overall circulatory health.

The emphasis on heart and circulatory health is not incidental. Modern lifestyles, characterized by high-stress environments, sedentary habits, and processed diets, have contributed to a rise in cardiovascular diseases. These conditions, often silent and progressive, can have severe implications if not addressed. Herbal approaches, coupled with lifestyle modifications, offer a proactive way to support and enhance cardiovascular health.

Herbs have been used for centuries to treat various health conditions, and their role in supporting heart health is significant. Many herbs are known for their cardiovascular benefits, including their ability to manage blood pressure and cholesterol levels and improve circulation. These natural remedies provide a gentler alternative to conventional treatments, often with fewer side effects. They work not just on symptoms but also address underlying causes and help in the overall strengthening of the heart and blood vessels.

Managing Blood Pressure:

High blood pressure, or hypertension, is a common condition that can lead to serious health problems like heart disease and stroke. The first part of this chapter focuses on herbal approaches to managing blood pressure. Herbs like hawthorn, garlic, and dandelion are highlighted for their ability to support cardiovascular health. These herbs can help relax blood vessels, improve blood flow, and support the heart's functioning.

For instance, hawthorn has been traditionally used to treat heart conditions and is known for its ability to strengthen the heart muscle, increase blood flow, and stabilize blood pressure. A tea made from hawthorn berries, leaves, or flowers can be a beneficial addition to a heart-healthy lifestyle.

Garlic, a common kitchen ingredient, has been shown to have a positive effect on blood pressure and cholesterol levels. It can be incorporated into the diet or taken in supplement form. Garlic's ability to thin the blood and reduce arterial plaque is also beneficial for overall circulatory health.

Cholesterol Management:

The second part of the chapter addresses cholesterol management, a key aspect of maintaining heart health. High levels of bad cholesterol (LDL) and low levels of good cholesterol (HDL) can lead to the buildup of plaque in arteries, increasing the risk of heart disease. Natural remedies for cholesterol management include dietary herbs and lifestyle tips that can help balance cholesterol levels.

Herbs like artichoke leaf extract, red yeast rice, and guggul have been found effective in managing cholesterol levels. Artichoke leaf extract, for instance, can help improve liver function and lower LDL cholesterol levels. It can be taken as a supplement or as a tea.

Dietary adjustments play a significant role in cholesterol management. Incorporating fiber-rich foods, omega-3 fatty acids, and healthy fats into the diet can help reduce cholesterol levels. Foods like oats, flaxseeds, nuts, and fatty fish are beneficial for heart health.

Circulatory Support:

The final part of the chapter focuses on supporting circulatory health. Good circulation is essential for transporting nutrients and oxygen throughout the body and removing waste products. Herbs like ginger, ginkgo biloba, and cayenne pepper are known for their ability to improve blood flow and support circulatory health.

Ginger, for example, has anti-inflammatory properties and can help improve blood circulation. It can be consumed as a fresh root, in powdered form, or as a tea. Ginkgo biloba, another powerful herb, is known for its ability to enhance blood flow to the brain and extremities, making it beneficial for overall circulatory health.

In addition to herbal remedies, this chapter emphasizes the importance of regular physical activity, maintaining a healthy weight, and managing stress for optimal heart and circulatory health. Simple practices like regular walking, yoga, and mindfulness techniques can have a profound impact on cardiovascular health.

In summary, Chapter 3 provides a detailed exploration of natural methods to support heart and circulatory health. It combines time-tested herbal remedies with practical lifestyle advice, offering a holistic approach to maintaining and enhancing cardiovascular health. This chapter serves as a guide to embracing natural solutions for heart health, encouraging readers to take proactive steps towards a healthier, more vibrant life.

BLOOD PRESSURE MANAGEMENT - HERBAL APPROACHES.

Managing blood pressure is a vital aspect of maintaining heart health and preventing a range of cardiovascular diseases. This subchapter presents a comprehensive approach to blood pressure management through the use of various herbs known for their cardiovascular benefits. The aim is to provide practical, natural solutions that can be integrated into daily life to support heart health and regulate blood pressure.

High blood pressure, or hypertension, is often referred to as a 'silent killer' because it typically has no symptoms but significantly increases the risk of heart disease and stroke. A combination of lifestyle changes and natural remedies can be incredibly effective in managing blood pressure. Herbs, with their multitude of medicinal properties, play a crucial role in this holistic approach.

Herbal Remedies for Blood Pressure Management:

- Hawthorn Berry Tea: Hawthorn berry has been used for centuries to treat heart and vascular diseases. It is known for its ability to strengthen the heart and blood vessels and improve circulation. Hawthorn berry tea can be made by steeping dried hawthorn berries in boiling water for about 10 minutes. Drinking this tea daily can help regulate blood pressure and support overall cardiovascular health.

- Garlic: Garlic is renowned for its health benefits, particularly for heart health. It helps to lower blood pressure by relaxing blood vessels and improving blood flow. Garlic can be incorporated into the diet in various forms - fresh, dried, or as a supplement. For those who prefer not to consume fresh garlic, odorless garlic capsules are available and can be taken as directed.

- Celery Seed Extract: Celery seed is a diuretic and vasodilator, making it useful in managing high blood pressure. It helps to increase urine output and relax blood vessel walls, thereby reducing blood pressure. Celery seed can be consumed as an extract or in its natural form. Adding celery to juices or meals is also a beneficial way to incorporate it into the diet.

- Dandelion Leaf Tea: Dandelion leaves are a natural diuretic, which can help in managing blood pressure by reducing fluid retention. To prepare dandelion leaf tea, steep dried leaves in boiling water for about 10 minutes. This tea can be consumed two to three times a day.

- Olive Leaf Extract: Olive leaf has been found to have a significant impact on lowering blood pressure. It can be consumed in the form of a supplement or as a tea. Olive leaf tea can be made by steeping dried olive leaves in hot water for several minutes.

Dietary and Lifestyle Tips for Blood Pressure Management:

Alongside these herbal remedies, certain dietary and lifestyle changes can greatly enhance blood pressure management.

- Reduce Sodium Intake: High sodium intake is linked to high blood pressure. Reducing salt in the diet can help manage blood pressure levels. Focus on eating fresh, whole foods and avoid processed foods high in sodium.
- Increase Potassium Intake: Potassium helps balance the amount of sodium in the cells and eases tension in the blood vessel walls. Foods rich in potassium include bananas, oranges, sweet potatoes, and spinach.
- Regular Physical Activity: Regular exercise strengthens the heart, allowing it to pump blood with less effort, which in turn lowers the pressure in the arteries. Aim for at least 30 minutes of moderate exercise, such as

brisk walking, swimming, or cycling, most days of the week.

- Maintain a Healthy Weight: Being overweight can increase the risk of high blood pressure. Losing even a small amount of weight if you're overweight or obese can help reduce blood pressure.
- Manage Stress: Chronic stress can contribute to high blood pressure. Techniques such as deep breathing, meditation, yoga, or tai chi can be effective in reducing stress levels.
- Limit Alcohol and Avoid Smoking: Excessive alcohol can raise blood pressure over time, while smoking damages blood vessels and raises the risk for high blood pressure.

In summary, this subchapter offers a range of herbal remedies and lifestyle tips for managing blood pressure. These natural approaches focus on supporting heart health and maintaining healthy blood pressure levels. Incorporating these remedies and habits into your daily routine can lead to significant improvements in blood pressure management and overall heart health. Remember, consistency is key in managing blood pressure, and these natural strategies should be part of a long-term approach to heart health.

CHOLESTEROL MANAGEMENT - NATURAL REMEDIES AND LIFESTYLE TIPS.

Cholesterol management is a critical aspect of maintaining heart health and reducing the risk of cardiovascular diseases. This subchapter is dedicated to exploring natural remedies and lifestyle changes that can effectively manage cholesterol levels.

High cholesterol, particularly low-density lipoprotein (LDL) or 'bad' cholesterol, can lead to the buildup of plaque in the arteries, increasing the risk of heart attack and stroke. The focus here is on practical, natural approaches to reducing LDL cholesterol and increasing high-density lipoprotein (HDL) or 'good' cholesterol.

Cholesterol management is not just about reducing numbers. It's about making sustainable changes to diet and lifestyle that can lead to long-term heart health. This holistic approach includes the use of dietary herbs, adjustments in eating habits, and lifestyle modifications.

Herbal Remedies for Cholesterol Management:

- Red Yeast Rice: Red yeast rice has compounds that can help reduce LDL cholesterol. It's made by fermenting a type of yeast called Monascus purpureus over red rice. Red yeast rice supplements are available and can be taken as directed. However, it is important to consult with a healthcare provider before starting any supplement, as red yeast rice can interact with certain medications.

- Artichoke Leaf Extract: Artichoke leaf has been found to lower cholesterol levels by inhibiting the synthesis of cholesterol in the body. Artichoke leaf extract is available in capsule form and can be a part of your cholesterol-lowering regimen.

- Green Tea: Green tea is rich in catechins and other antioxidants that can help lower LDL cholesterol and improve HDL cholesterol. Incorporating green tea into your daily routine can be a simple yet effective way to manage cholesterol. Aim for two to three cups per day for the best results.

- Garlic: Garlic is known for its cholesterol-lowering properties. It can be included in the diet or taken in the form of supplements. Garlic not only helps lower LDL cholesterol but also has a positive effect on overall heart health.

- Fenugreek Seeds: Fenugreek seeds contain saponins, which can help reduce the body's absorption of cholesterol from fatty foods. These seeds can be soaked overnight and consumed in the morning, or can be powdered and added to food.

Dietary Adjustments for Cholesterol Management:

Diet plays a crucial role in managing cholesterol levels. Incorporating certain foods into your diet while reducing or eliminating others can make a significant difference.

- Fiber-Rich Foods: Soluble fiber can reduce the absorption of cholesterol in the bloodstream. Foods high in soluble fiber include oats, barley, beans, lentils, apples, and pears.
- Omega-3 Fatty Acids: Omega-3 fatty acids are known to reduce triglycerides, a type of fat in the blood, and

increase HDL cholesterol. Foods rich in omega-3s include fatty fish like salmon, mackerel, and sardines, as well as flaxseeds and walnuts.

- Nuts and Seeds: Nuts and seeds are excellent sources of healthy fats and can help reduce LDL cholesterol. Almonds, walnuts, flaxseeds, and chia seeds are great choices to include in your diet.
- Plant Sterols and Stanols: These substances, found in plants, help block the absorption of cholesterol. They are added to certain foods like margarines, orange juice, and yogurt drinks.
- Reduce Saturated and Trans Fats: Reducing the intake of saturated fats found in red meat and full-fat dairy products, as well as eliminating trans fats found in partially hydrogenated oils, is crucial for cholesterol management.

Lifestyle Tips for Cholesterol Management:

In addition to dietary changes, certain lifestyle modifications can also help manage cholesterol levels.

- Regular Exercise: Regular physical activity can help improve cholesterol levels. Aim for at least 30 minutes of moderate-intensity exercise most days of the week.
- Weight Management: Losing weight can help lower cholesterol levels. Even a small amount of weight loss can have a positive impact.
- Quitting Smoking: Smoking lowers HDL cholesterol and damages the walls of blood vessels, making them more susceptible to the accumulation of fatty deposits.

- Limit Alcohol Intake: Excessive alcohol consumption can raise cholesterol levels. It's important to drink in moderation.
- Stress Reduction: Chronic stress may contribute to higher cholesterol levels. Practices like meditation, yoga, and deep breathing can be effective in reducing stress.

In conclusion, managing cholesterol is not solely about taking medication. It involves a holistic approach that includes herbal remedies, dietary changes, and lifestyle modifications. These natural strategies work together to lower LDL cholesterol, raise HDL cholesterol, and promote overall heart health. By incorporating these changes into your daily life, you can effectively manage your cholesterol levels and reduce your risk of heart disease. Remember, consistency and a commitment to a healthier lifestyle are key to successful cholesterol management.

CIRCULATORY SUPPORT - ENHANCING BLOOD FLOW AND HEART HEALTH

Good circulation is fundamental to overall health. It is the circulatory system that delivers oxygen and nutrients to every cell in the body and removes waste products. This subchapter focuses on herbs and practices that support circulatory health, emphasizing natural ways to improve blood flow and maintain heart health.

Poor circulation can lead to various health issues, including fatigue, cold hands and feet, muscle cramps, and even heart problems. Enhancing circulation naturally is about more than just addressing these symptoms; it's about improving the overall functioning of the circulatory system. This can be achieved through a combination of herbal remedies, dietary adjustments, and lifestyle changes.

Herbal Remedies for Circulatory Support:

- Ginkgo Biloba: Ginkgo is well-known for its ability to improve blood flow, especially to the brain, making it beneficial for cognitive function. It works by dilating blood vessels and reducing the stickiness of blood platelets. To use ginkgo, you can take standardized extracts in capsule or tablet form. It's important to follow the dosage instructions, as ginkgo can interact with certain medications.

- Horse Chestnut: Horse chestnut is known for its effectiveness in reducing inflammation and strengthening the walls of blood vessels, making it particularly useful for varicose veins and chronic venous insufficiency. The active compound in horse chestnut is aescin, which helps tighten the veins and prevent fluid leakage. Horse chestnut can be taken as a capsule, extract, or tea.

- Cayenne Pepper: Cayenne pepper is a powerful circulatory stimulant. It helps to increase blood flow, strengthen arteries and capillaries, and reduce blood cholesterol and triglyceride levels. Cayenne can be included in the diet or taken as a supplement in capsule form.

- Hawthorn Berry: Hawthorn is a heart tonic that helps improve circulation, strengthen the heart, and stabilize heart rhythm. It can be taken as a tea, tincture, or in capsule form. Hawthorn is especially beneficial for those with heart failure, angina, or hypertension.

- Ginger: Ginger is another herb that promotes circulation. It can be added to food, taken as a supplement, or consumed as a tea. Ginger helps to warm the body and improve blood flow, making it beneficial for those with poor circulation.

Dietary Changes for Better Circulation:

Diet plays a crucial role in circulatory health. Certain foods can help improve circulation and support heart health.

- Omega-3 Fatty Acids: Omega-3s are essential for heart health. They help to reduce blood pressure and inflammation, which can improve circulation. Foods rich in omega-3s include salmon, mackerel, walnuts, and flaxseeds.
- Dark Chocolate: Rich in flavonoids, dark chocolate can improve circulation. It's important to choose chocolate with a high cocoa content and consume it in moderation.
- Berries: Berries, such as blueberries, raspberries, and strawberries, are high in antioxidants and can help improve blood flow and support overall heart health.

- Leafy Greens: Leafy greens like spinach and kale are high in nitrates, which the body converts into nitric oxide, a molecule that helps improve blood flow.

Lifestyle Practices for Circulatory Health:

In addition to herbal remedies and diet, certain lifestyle practices can significantly improve circulation.

- Regular Exercise: Physical activity is one of the best ways to improve circulation. Activities like walking, jogging, swimming, and cycling help strengthen the heart and improve blood flow.
- Hydration: Staying well-hydrated is essential for good circulation. Water helps thin the blood, making it easier for it to flow through the vessels.
- Elevating Legs: For those with poor leg circulation, elevating the legs can help reduce swelling and improve blood flow.
- Massage and Hydrotherapy: Massage and water therapies can stimulate blood flow. Techniques like dry brushing or taking contrast showers (alternating between hot and cold water) can be particularly effective.
- Avoiding Tight Clothing: Tight clothing, especially around the waist or legs, can restrict blood flow. Wearing loose, comfortable clothing can help improve circulation.
- Quitting Smoking: Smoking contributes to the narrowing and hardening of the arteries, reducing blood flow. Quitting smoking is crucial for improving circulatory health.

In conclusion, this subchapter offers a holistic approach to improving circulatory health, combining herbal remedies, dietary advice, and lifestyle changes. By incorporating these practices into your daily routine, you can significantly enhance blood flow and support your heart health. Remember, the key to good circulation is a combination of a healthy diet, regular physical activity, and natural remedies that support the vascular system.

CHAPTER 4: SKIN CARE AND DERMATOLOGICAL HEALTH.

Chapter 4 is devoted to skin care and dermatological health, a vital aspect of our overall well-being. Skin, the largest organ of the body, is often a reflection of our internal health and is subject to a variety of conditions that can affect its appearance and function. In this chapter, we delve into natural and holistic approaches to skin care, focusing on herbal remedies for common skin conditions like acne and eczema, psoriasis and skin rashes, and providing DIY herbal skincare recipes suitable for everyday use.

The skin is not just a protective barrier; it's a dynamic organ with complex functions, including regulation of temperature and synthesis of vitamin D. Its health is influenced by various factors such as genetics, diet, lifestyle, and environmental exposures. Common skin conditions like acne, eczema, and psoriasis not only affect physical appearance but can also lead to discomfort and impact mental well-being. Conventional treatments for these conditions often include harsh chemicals or medications that may have undesirable side effects. This chapter introduces a gentler, more natural approach to skin care, harnessing the power of herbs known for their healing, anti-inflammatory, and soothing properties.

Holistic Approach to Skin Care:

The holistic approach to skin care acknowledges that skin health is intricately linked to overall health. Factors such as diet, hydration, stress, sleep, and gut health significantly impact skin condition. A diet rich in antioxidants, omega-3 fatty acids, vitamins, and minerals can promote healthy skin. Adequate hydration ensures that the skin remains supple and helps in the detoxification process. Managing stress through relaxation techniques and ensuring sufficient sleep are also crucial for maintaining skin health. Additionally, gut health, influenced by diet and probiotics, plays a key role in skin condition, as imbalances in gut flora can manifest as skin issues.

Natural Remedies for Common Skin Conditions:

Herbal remedies offer a natural way to manage skin conditions by reducing inflammation, soothing irritation, and promoting healing. For acne, herbs such as tea tree, neem, and turmeric offer antibacterial and anti-inflammatory properties. Eczema, characterized by dry, itchy, and inflamed skin, can be soothed with herbs like chamomile, calendula, and oatmeal, which have healing and calming effects. Psoriasis, involving red, scaly patches on the skin, can be managed with aloe vera, Oregon grape, and evening primrose oil, known for their skin-reparative qualities.

DIY Herbal Skincare:

This chapter also includes a section on DIY herbal skincare recipes. These recipes are designed to be simple, effective, and adaptable for different skin types. They utilize common herbs and natural ingredients to create cleansers, toners, moisturizers, and masks. The emphasis is on using pure, organic ingredients to nourish and rejuvenate the skin without exposure to harmful chemicals commonly found in commercial skincare products.

Practical Tips for Skin Health:

In addition to herbal remedies, this chapter offers practical tips for maintaining skin health. These include advice on gentle cleansing, avoiding overexposure to the sun, and choosing natural, non-comedogenic (non-pore-clogging) skincare products. Tips on lifestyle changes, such as reducing sugar intake and avoiding dairy products, which can exacerbate certain skin conditions, are also discussed.

This chapter did provide a comprehensive guide to natural skin care and the management of common skin conditions. It highlights the importance of a holistic approach to skin health, considering both external treatments and internal factors. By adopting the practices and remedies outlined in this chapter, readers can enjoy healthier, more radiant skin and improve their overall well-being. The focus is on empowering individuals with the knowledge and tools to care for their skin naturally and effectively, embracing the beauty and benefits of herbal wisdom.

ACNE AND ECZEMA - HERBAL REMEDIES.

Acne and eczema are two prevalent skin conditions that affect a significant portion of the population. While they are distinct conditions, acne being characterized by pimples and blocked pores, and eczema by dry, itchy, and inflamed skin; both can be addressed effectively with herbal remedies. This subchapter focuses on providing practical, detailed recipes for treating acne and eczema, emphasizing the use of anti-inflammatory and skin-healing herbs.

Herbal Remedies for Acne:

Acne, often a result of clogged pores, bacteria, and inflammation, can be a source of discomfort and self-consciousness. Herbal treatments for acne focus on reducing inflammation, combating bacterial growth, and promoting skin healing.

- Tea Tree Oil Application: Tea tree oil is renowned for its antibacterial and anti-inflammatory properties, making it an excellent treatment for acne. To use, mix a few drops of tea tree oil with a carrier oil like jojoba or sweet almond oil to dilute it, and apply it directly to the affected areas using a cotton swab. Be careful to avoid the surrounding skin, as tea tree oil can be quite potent.

- Green Tea Toner: Green tea, rich in antioxidants, can reduce inflammation and sebum production in acne-prone skin. Brew a strong cup of green tea and let it cool. Use a clean cloth or cotton pad to apply the tea to your face or just the acne-prone areas. Leave it on for a few minutes before rinsing.

- Neem and Honey Mask: Neem has antibacterial properties that are effective in treating acne. Mix neem powder with raw honey to form a paste. Apply this mask to the face, focusing on acne-prone areas, and leave it on for about 20 minutes before rinsing with warm water.

- Aloe Vera Gel: Aloe vera is soothing and anti-inflammatory, ideal for reducing the redness and swelling associated with acne. Apply pure aloe vera gel to the skin and let it sit for 30 minutes before rinsing. This can be done daily.

Herbal Remedies for Eczema:

Eczema, characterized by dry, itchy, and inflamed skin, can be treated with herbs that have moisturizing and anti-inflammatory properties.

- Oatmeal Bath: Oatmeal has soothing properties that are beneficial for eczema-prone skin. Add a cup of colloidal oatmeal to a warm bath and soak for 15-20 minutes. This helps to soothe itchiness and irritation.

- Calendula Cream: Calendula is known for its healing and anti-inflammatory properties. To make a calendula cream, infuse calendula petals in a carrier oil like coconut or olive oil. Strain and mix the infused oil with shea butter to create a moisturizing cream. Apply this to the affected areas a few times a day.

- Chamomile Compress: Chamomile is soothing and can reduce inflammation in eczema-prone skin. Brew a strong chamomile tea, let it cool, and then use a clean cloth to apply it as a compress to the irritated skin.

- Witch Hazel Toner: Witch hazel has astringent properties, which can help soothe eczema. Apply witch hazel with a cotton ball to the affected areas. Ensure that you use a non-alcoholic witch hazel extract to avoid skin dryness.

Lifestyle and Dietary Tips:

In addition to these remedies, certain lifestyle and dietary changes can enhance skin health:

- Hydration: Keep the skin hydrated by drinking plenty of water and using a humidifier in dry environments.
- Gentle Skincare Products: Use gentle, fragrance-free skincare products to avoid irritation.
- Balanced Diet: Eat a diet rich in omega-3 fatty acids, antioxidants, and vitamins, which can help improve skin health. Foods like fatty fish, nuts, seeds, and leafy greens are beneficial.
- Stress Management: Stress can exacerbate both acne and eczema. Practices like yoga, meditation, and regular exercise can help manage stress levels.
- Avoid Trigger Foods: Certain foods can trigger or worsen acne and eczema. Common triggers include dairy, gluten, and refined sugars. Keep a food diary to identify and avoid potential trigger foods.

In summary, this subchapter offers a range of herbal remedies and practical tips for managing acne and eczema. These natural approaches focus on reducing inflammation, soothing irritation, and promoting skin healing. By incorporating these remedies and lifestyle adjustments into your daily routine, you can effectively manage these skin conditions and improve your overall skin health. Remember, consistency and patience are key, as natural remedies may take time to show results.

PSORIASIS AND SKIN RASHES - NATURAL TREATMENTS.

Psoriasis and skin rashes can be persistent and uncomfortable conditions, affecting not just the physical aspect of skin but also impacting emotional well-being. This subchapter is dedicated to natural treatments for these skin issues, focusing on both topical applications and internal remedies to alleviate symptoms and promote healing. Psoriasis, characterized by red, scaly patches on the skin, and various types of skin rashes, each demand a unique approach to treatment. The remedies provided here are grounded in the understanding that skin health is deeply connected to overall wellness.

Natural Remedies for Psoriasis:

Psoriasis is a chronic condition that often requires a multifaceted approach to treatment. These natural remedies aim to soothe irritated skin, reduce inflammation, and support the body's healing processes.

- Turmeric: Turmeric, with its active compound curcumin, is known for its anti-inflammatory properties. It can be effective in reducing psoriasis flare-ups. For a topical application, make a paste by mixing turmeric powder with a bit of water and apply it to the affected areas. Internally, turmeric can be included in the diet or taken as a supplement.

- Aloe Vera Gel: Aloe vera is soothing and moisturizing, making it an excellent remedy for the dry, itchy skin associated with psoriasis. Apply pure aloe vera gel to the affected areas to reduce redness and itching. The gel can be extracted directly from an aloe vera plant or purchased in its pure form.

- Apple Cider Vinegar: Diluted apple cider vinegar can help alleviate scalp psoriasis. Mix equal parts of apple cider vinegar and water and apply it to the scalp. Rinse thoroughly after a few minutes. Avoid this remedy if there are open wounds or cracks in the skin.

- Oatmeal Bath: An oatmeal bath can provide relief from itching and redness. Grind plain oatmeal into a fine powder and add it to a lukewarm bath. Soaking in this bath can help soothe psoriasis symptoms.

- Tea Tree Oil: Known for its antiseptic properties, tea tree oil can help reduce the risk of infection in psoriatic skin lesions. Mix a few drops of tea tree oil with a carrier oil like coconut oil and apply it to the affected areas.

Natural Treatments for Skin Rashes:

Skin rashes can be caused by a variety of factors, including allergies, infections, or environmental irritants. The following remedies are geared toward soothing the skin, reducing inflammation, and promoting healing.

- Chamomile Compress: Chamomile has anti-inflammatory and soothing properties, making it ideal for treating skin rashes. Brew a strong chamomile tea, let it cool, and then use a clean cloth to apply it to the rash as a compress.

- Calendula Cream: Calendula is effective in healing and soothing irritated skin. You can make a homemade calendula cream by infusing calendula petals in a carrier oil, straining the mixture, and then blending it with beeswax to create a thick cream.

- Witch Hazel: Witch hazel is a natural astringent that can help relieve itching and irritation. Apply witch hazel extract directly to the rash with a cotton ball.
- Coconut Oil: Coconut oil is moisturizing and has anti-inflammatory properties. It can be particularly helpful for rashes caused by dry skin. Apply virgin coconut oil directly to the rash several times a day.

- Baking Soda Bath: Baking soda can help reduce itching and inflammation associated with rashes. Add a cup of baking soda to a bathtub filled with cool water and soak for about 15-20 minutes.

Dietary and Lifestyle Tips for Skin Health:

In addition to topical treatments, dietary and lifestyle changes can significantly impact the management of psoriasis and skin rashes.

- Anti-Inflammatory Diet: An anti-inflammatory diet can help reduce psoriasis flare-ups and skin inflammation. This includes consuming plenty of fruits, vegetables, whole grains, lean proteins, and omega-3 fatty acids.
- Hydration: Adequate hydration is key for maintaining healthy skin. Ensure you drink enough water throughout the day.
- Avoid Trigger Foods: Certain foods can exacerbate psoriasis and skin rashes. Common triggers include alcohol, red meat, and processed foods.
- Stress Management: Stress can trigger or worsen psoriasis and other skin conditions. Engage in stress-reducing activities such as yoga, meditation, or regular exercise.
- Sun Exposure: Moderate sun exposure can improve psoriasis symptoms, but it's important to avoid sunburn. Always use a broad-spectrum sunscreen and limit your time in direct sunlight.

In conclusion, this subchapter provides a comprehensive guide to managing psoriasis and skin rashes using natural remedies. These treatments, combined with appropriate dietary and lifestyle changes, offer a holistic approach to skin health. The emphasis is on gentle, natural ingredients that soothe and heal the skin while addressing underlying causes of skin conditions. Adopting these practices can lead to noticeable improvements in skin health and overall well-being.

Herbal Skincare Recipes – Tailored for Every Skin Type.

In the realm of natural skincare, the use of herbs and organic ingredients plays a pivotal role in nurturing and maintaining the skin's health and radiance. This subchapter is dedicated to DIY herbal skincare recipes, offering a variety of formulations tailored for different skin types. These recipes provide practical, natural solutions for everyday skincare, harnessing the therapeutic properties of herbs to address various skin needs and concerns.

Creating your own skincare products not only allows you to tailor ingredients to your specific skin type but also ensures that you are using fresh, natural, and chemical-free ingredients on your skin. Whether you have oily, dry, combination, sensitive, or mature skin, these recipes can be adapted to suit your individual needs.

1. Herbal Cleanser for Oily Skin:

Oily skin requires a gentle cleanser that can remove excess oil without stripping the skin of its natural oils.

- Ingredients: Green tea, honey, apple cider vinegar, and castile soap.
- Recipe: Brew a strong cup of green tea and let it cool. Mix 1/4 cup of green tea with 1 tablespoon of raw honey, 1 tablespoon of apple cider vinegar, and 1/4 cup of liquid castile soap. Store in a pump bottle and use daily.

2. Nourishing Face Cream for Dry Skin:

Dry skin needs extra nourishment and hydration, which can be provided by rich, moisturizing ingredients.

- Ingredients: Shea butter, almond oil, coconut oil, and lavender essential oil.
- Recipe: Melt 1/2 cup of shea butter, 1/4 cup of almond oil, and 1/4 cup of coconut oil in a double boiler. Once melted, remove from heat and let it cool slightly. Add 10-15 drops of lavender essential oil and whisk until creamy. Store in a jar and use as needed.

3. Toning Facial Mist for Combination Skin:

Combination skin benefits from a balancing toner that can hydrate dry areas while controlling oil in the T-zone.

- Ingredients: Rose water, witch hazel, and geranium essential oil.
- Recipe: Mix 1/2 cup of rose water with 1/4 cup of witch hazel and 5 drops of geranium essential oil. Pour into a spray bottle and use as a refreshing toner after cleansing.

4. Gentle Exfoliating Scrub for Sensitive Skin:

Sensitive skin requires a gentle exfoliant that can remove dead skin cells without causing irritation.

- Ingredients: Oatmeal, honey, and yogurt.
- Recipe: Grind 1/4 cup of oatmeal into a fine powder. Mix with 2 tablespoons of honey and 2 tablespoons of yogurt to form a paste. Gently massage onto the face, then rinse off with warm water.

5. Anti-Aging Serum for Mature Skin:

Mature skin benefits from ingredients that are rich in antioxidants and have anti-aging properties.

- Ingredients: Argan oil, rosehip oil, and frankincense essential oil.
- Recipe: Mix 1/4 cup of argan oil with 1/4 cup of rosehip oil and add 10 drops of frankincense essential oil. Store in a dark glass bottle and apply a few drops to the face and neck before bedtime.

6. Soothing Herbal Mask for All Skin Types:

A soothing herbal mask can benefit all skin types by calming the skin and providing essential nutrients.

- Ingredients: Chamomile, aloe vera gel, and green clay.

- Recipe: Steep 2 chamomile tea bags in hot water, then let the tea cool. Mix 1/4 cup of the chamomile tea with 2 tablespoons of aloe vera gel and enough green clay to form a paste. Apply to the face and leave on for 10-15 minutes before rinsing off.

Lifestyle and Dietary Tips for Skin Health:

In addition to these topical applications, maintaining skin health also involves lifestyle and dietary choices:

- Stay Hydrated: Drinking plenty of water is essential for maintaining skin hydration.
- Balanced Diet: Eating a diet rich in fruits, vegetables, lean proteins, and healthy fats provides the nutrients needed for healthy skin.
- Sun Protection: Protecting the skin from excessive sun exposure is crucial to prevent damage and premature aging. Use a broad-spectrum sunscreen when outdoors.
- Adequate Sleep: Ensuring sufficient sleep helps in skin repair and regeneration.

In conclusion, this subchapter offers a range of DIY herbal skincare recipes tailored for various skin types, along with essential lifestyle and dietary tips. By incorporating these natural skincare solutions into your routine, you can achieve healthier, more radiant skin. These recipes emphasize the beauty of simplicity and the effectiveness of natural ingredients, providing a wholesome approach to skincare.

Chapter 5: Joint and Muscle Health.

Chapter 5 takes a close look at joint and muscle health, areas of the body that are integral to our mobility and overall well-being. This chapter is devoted to understanding and addressing common issues such as arthritis, joint pain, muscle aches, and strains through natural and holistic approaches. It also delves into the therapeutic benefits of soothing herbal baths, which can provide significant relief and relaxation.

Joint and muscle health is crucial at every stage of life. Whether due to the natural aging process, an active lifestyle, or specific conditions like arthritis, joint and muscle discomfort can greatly impact quality of life. Traditional treatments for these ailments often include medications that can have side effects or fail to address the root cause of the discomfort. In contrast, the natural remedies and lifestyle tips provided in this chapter offer a gentler and more holistic approach to managing joint and muscle health.

Understanding Joint and Muscle Health:

Joints are the connections between bones, providing support and helping us move. Any damage to the joints from disease or injury can interfere with movement and cause pain. Arthritis, one of the most common causes of joint pain, encompasses a range of joint diseases and conditions. Similarly, muscle health is vital for movement, balance, and strength. Muscle aches and strains can result from overuse, tension, or injuries.

The body's ability to heal and maintain joint and muscle health can be significantly enhanced through natural means. This includes the use of herbal remedies known for their anti-inflammatory, analgesic, and healing properties, as well as lifestyle adjustments that support joint and muscle function.

Herbal Approaches to Arthritis and Joint Pain:

Arthritis and joint pain can be managed effectively with herbs that possess anti-inflammatory and pain-relieving properties. These herbs can be used in various forms, such as teas, tinctures, oils, or topical applications.

- Turmeric and Ginger Tea: Both turmeric and ginger contain compounds with potent anti-inflammatory properties, making them excellent for joint pain relief. Regular consumption of tea made from these herbs can help reduce inflammation and alleviate pain.

- Willow Bark: Often referred to as "nature's aspirin," willow bark has been used for centuries to relieve pain and inflammation. It can be taken as a tea or in a capsule form to help ease arthritis and joint pain.

- Eucalyptus Oil: Eucalyptus oil has natural pain-relieving and anti-inflammatory properties. Applying diluted eucalyptus oil topically to painful joints can provide relief.

- Nettle Leaf: Nettle leaf, when taken as a tea or supplement, can help reduce inflammation and pain associated with arthritis.

Remedies for Muscle Aches and Strains:

Muscle aches and strains can benefit from herbal treatments that promote relaxation, reduce muscle tension, and alleviate pain.

- Arnica: Arnica is known for its ability to reduce pain and swelling associated with muscle strains. Arnica creams or gels can be applied topically to affected areas.

- Comfrey: Comfrey has compounds that help reduce muscle pain and accelerate healing. A poultice made from comfrey leaves can be applied to sore muscles for relief.

- Magnesium-rich Herbal Baths: Soaking in a bath infused with Epsom salts, which are high in magnesium, can help relax muscle aches. Herbs like lavender or chamomile can be added for extra relaxation benefits.

Soothing Herbal Baths for Overall Relief:

Herbal baths can provide comprehensive relief from joint and muscle pain, along with promoting relaxation and stress relief.

- Lavender and Epsom Salt Bath: A bath with Epsom salts and lavender essential oil can soothe sore muscles and joints, reduce stress, and promote better sleep.

- Rosemary and Peppermint Bath: Rosemary and peppermint have natural anti-inflammatory and analgesic properties. Adding these herbs or their essential oils to a warm bath can help alleviate muscle stiffness and joint pain.

- Chamomile Bath: Chamomile is known for its calming properties. A chamomile-infused bath can help reduce inflammation and soothe muscle and joint discomfort.

Lifestyle Tips for Joint and Muscle Health:

In addition to herbal remedies, certain lifestyle changes can significantly improve joint and muscle health:

- Regular Exercise: Regular, moderate exercise can strengthen muscles, improve joint flexibility, and reduce pain.
- Healthy Diet: A diet rich in anti-inflammatory foods like omega-3 fatty acids, antioxidants, and fiber can support joint and muscle health.

- Adequate Hydration: Staying hydrated helps maintain the health of the joint's synovial fluid, which reduces friction and enables smooth joint movement.
- Weight Management: Maintaining a healthy weight reduces the strain on joints, particularly in the knees, hips, and back.

In summary, Chapter 5 provides a detailed exploration of natural and holistic methods for managing joint and muscle health. Through a combination of herbal remedies, dietary recommendations, and lifestyle changes, this chapter offers a comprehensive approach to improving joint and muscle function, enhancing mobility, and reducing pain and discomfort. Adopting these practices can lead to significant improvements in joint and muscle health, contributing to a better quality of life and overall well-being.

ARTHRITIS AND JOINT PAIN - MANAGING WITH HERBAL REMEDIES AND LIFESTYLE CHANGES.

Arthritis and joint pain, common ailments that affect many, can significantly hinder daily activities and quality of life. This subchapter focuses on providing detailed herbal recipes and lifestyle tips to manage and alleviate the symptoms associated with these conditions. Arthritis, characterized by inflammation, pain, and stiffness in the joints, can be addressed through a combination of natural remedies and lifestyle modifications that aim to reduce inflammation, alleviate pain, and enhance joint mobility.

Herbal Remedies for Arthritis and Joint Pain:

The use of herbs in managing arthritis and joint pain is rooted in their anti-inflammatory and analgesic properties. These remedies offer a natural alternative to conventional pain relievers, targeting the inflammation and pain associated with arthritis.

- Turmeric and Ginger Capsules: Both turmeric and ginger are renowned for their anti-inflammatory properties. They can be taken in capsule form for ease of use and dosage control. To make your own capsules, mix equal parts of turmeric and ginger powder. Using a capsule machine, fill empty capsules with this mixture. Take 1-2 capsules twice daily with meals. Note: It's important to consult with a healthcare provider before starting any new supplement, especially if you are on medication or have health concerns.

- Rosehip and Nettle Tea: Rosehip is rich in vitamin C and antioxidants, while nettle is known for its anti-inflammatory properties. To make this tea, mix dried rosehip and nettle leaves in equal parts. Steep one teaspoon of this blend in hot water for about 10 minutes. Drink this tea twice a day to help reduce inflammation and joint pain.

- Eucalyptus Oil Rub: Eucalyptus oil has natural anti-inflammatory properties. Mix a few drops of eucalyptus oil with a carrier oil like coconut oil and massage it into the affected joints. This can help reduce pain and inflammation.

- Boswellia Serrata Supplement: Also known as Indian frankincense, Boswellia serrata has been shown to reduce inflammation and can be effective in treating arthritis. Boswellia supplements are available in health stores. Follow the dosage instructions on the product, and consult with a healthcare provider before starting any new supplement.

Lifestyle Tips for Managing Arthritis and Joint Pain:

In addition to herbal remedies, lifestyle changes can play a significant role in managing arthritis and joint pain.

- Regular Exercise: Low-impact exercises such as walking, swimming, or yoga can help maintain joint flexibility and strength without putting excessive strain on the joints.
- Healthy Diet: Incorporate anti-inflammatory foods into your diet. Foods rich in omega-3 fatty acids (like salmon and flaxseeds), antioxidants (like berries and leafy greens), and spices (like turmeric and ginger) can help reduce inflammation.
- Maintain a Healthy Weight: Extra weight can put additional pressure on joints, particularly the knees, hips, and spine. Losing weight can help reduce this stress and alleviate pain.
- Hot and Cold Therapy: Applying heat to stiff joints can help increase blood flow and relax muscles. Cold treatments, like ice packs, can reduce joint swelling and pain.

- Stress Management: Chronic stress can worsen arthritis symptoms. Techniques such as deep breathing, meditation, or tai chi can help manage stress levels.
- Adequate Rest: Ensure you get enough sleep, as rest is crucial for the body's healing process. Using ergonomic and supportive pillows can also help reduce joint pain during sleep.
- Stay Hydrated: Proper hydration is important for joint lubrication. Aim to drink at least 8 glasses of water a day.

In conclusion, this subchapter provides a comprehensive approach to managing arthritis and joint pain through natural herbal remedies and lifestyle modifications. These strategies are aimed at reducing inflammation, alleviating pain, and improving joint function. By incorporating these remedies and changes into your daily routine, you can effectively manage arthritis symptoms and enhance your overall joint health. Remember, consistency is key, and it's important to listen to your body and adjust these practices according to your individual needs.

MUSCLE ACHES AND STRAINS - HERBAL REMEDIES AND SOOTHING PRACTICES.

Muscle aches and strains are common ailments that can arise from various causes such as physical activity, stress, or underlying health conditions. This subchapter is dedicated to providing practical and effective herbal remedies, including compresses and baths, to alleviate muscle discomfort. These natural approaches focus on relieving pain, reducing inflammation, and promoting muscle relaxation and recovery.

Muscular health is crucial for overall mobility and quality of life. When muscles are strained or overworked, the body often responds with pain and stiffness. While rest is essential, certain herbal treatments can significantly aid the healing process. These treatments are not only effective in alleviating pain but also in nurturing the muscles and surrounding tissues, promoting overall muscular health.

Herbal Compresses for Muscle Relief:

Herbal compresses are an excellent way to apply healing herbs directly to sore muscles. The warmth of the compress can also aid in increasing blood flow and reducing muscle spasms.

- Arnica and Comfrey Compress: Both arnica and comfrey are known for their pain-relieving and anti-inflammatory properties, making them ideal for treating muscle aches. To prepare a compress, steep arnica and comfrey leaves in hot water for 10 minutes. Soak a clean cloth in this infusion, wring out the excess water, and apply it to the affected area for 15-20 minutes. Repeat this process 2-3 times a day.

- Lavender and Chamomile Compress: Lavender and chamomile are soothing herbs that can help relax tense muscles. Make an infusion by steeping these herbs in boiling water. Apply the warm, moist cloth to sore areas to ease muscle tension.

Herbal Baths for Muscle Aches and Strains:

A warm bath infused with healing herbs can provide immense relief for muscle aches and strains. The combination of warm water and medicinal herbs helps to relax muscles, reduce pain, and promote a sense of well-being.

- Epsom Salt and Eucalyptus Bath: Epsom salt is rich in magnesium, which is essential for muscle function and can help relieve soreness. Add two cups of Epsom salt and 10-15 drops of eucalyptus oil to a warm bath. Soak for at least 20 minutes to allow the body to absorb the magnesium and benefit from the eucalyptus' pain-relieving properties.

- Rosemary and Ginger Bath: Rosemary and ginger both have anti-inflammatory properties, making them beneficial for muscle pain. Add a handful of rosemary leaves and a few slices of fresh ginger to a hot bath. Soaking in this bath can help alleviate muscle soreness and improve circulation.

Topical Herbal Remedies for Muscle Recovery:

Applying herbal remedies directly to the skin can provide targeted relief to sore muscles.

- Peppermint and Marjoram Oil Blend: Mix equal parts of peppermint and marjoram essential oils with a carrier oil like almond or jojoba oil. Massage this blend onto sore muscles for a cooling and soothing effect.

- Cayenne and Olive Oil Rub: Cayenne pepper contains capsaicin, a natural pain reliever. Mix a teaspoon of cayenne pepper with a cup of olive oil. Apply this mixture to the affected area, but be sure to avoid any open cuts or sensitive areas.

Internal Remedies for Supporting Muscle Health:

In addition to topical treatments, certain internal remedies can support muscle health and recovery.

- Turmeric and Black Pepper Capsules: Turmeric contains curcumin, a compound with potent anti-inflammatory properties. Taking turmeric capsules along with black pepper, which increases curcumin absorption, can help reduce internal inflammation and muscle pain.

- Cherry Juice: Tart cherry juice is known for its anti-inflammatory and antioxidant properties. Drinking tart cherry juice can help reduce muscle soreness, especially after exercise.

Lifestyle Tips for Preventing Muscle Aches and Strains:

Preventative measures are just as important as treatments when it comes to muscle health.

- Regular Stretching: Incorporating stretching into your daily routine can help maintain muscle flexibility and prevent strains.
- Adequate Hydration: Staying hydrated is essential for muscle health and can prevent cramps and strains.
- Balanced Diet: A diet rich in anti-inflammatory foods, protein, and essential vitamins and minerals supports muscle recovery and overall health.
- Proper Posture and Ergonomics: Maintaining good posture and using ergonomic tools can help prevent muscle strain, especially for those who sit for long periods.

In conclusion, this subchapter offers a comprehensive guide to managing muscle aches and strains through herbal remedies, soothing practices, and lifestyle changes. These natural strategies focus on relieving pain, reducing inflammation, and supporting muscle recovery, enhancing overall muscle health. By integrating these remedies and practices into your routine, you can effectively manage muscle discomfort and maintain healthy, functional muscles.

SOOTHING HERBAL BATHS - PAIN RELIEF AND RELAXATION RECIPES.

In the pursuit of holistic wellness, the ancient practice of herbal baths holds a special place, especially for those seeking relief from pain and stress. This subchapter is dedicated to exploring the art of creating soothing herbal baths. Each recipe is crafted to provide not just physical relief from pain and discomfort but also to offer a serene, meditative experience that nurtures the mind and soul.

Herbal baths harness the therapeutic properties of natural herbs, combined with the relaxing and restorative power of warm water. These baths can be particularly beneficial for individuals dealing with joint pain, muscle aches, stress, or simply looking for a natural way to unwind after a long day.

Introduction to Herbal Bath Preparations:

Creating an herbal bath involves more than just adding herbs to hot water. It's about understanding the properties of each herb and how they interact with the body and mind. The temperature of the water, the duration of the bath, and the combination of herbs all play a pivotal role in the effectiveness of the bath.

- Temperature Considerations: The ideal temperature for an herbal bath should be warm but not overly hot. Excessively hot water can cause skin irritation and may be detrimental to the therapeutic properties of some herbs.

- Duration of Bath: A typical herbal bath should last between 15 to 30 minutes. This duration allows enough time for the skin to absorb the beneficial properties of the herbs.

- Herb Selection: Choose herbs based on their therapeutic properties. For pain relief, herbs with anti-inflammatory and analgesic properties are ideal. For relaxation, herbs with calming and soothing properties should be selected.

Herbal Bath Recipes for Pain Relief and Relaxation:

Each of these recipes is designed to target specific needs, whether it's soothing sore muscles, calming an overactive mind, or rejuvenating tired skin.

- Muscle Relief Herbal Bath:
  - Ingredients: Epsom salt, lavender flowers, chamomile flowers, and rosemary leaves.
  - Recipe: Combine 2 cups of Epsom salt, 1/2 cup dried lavender flowers, 1/2 cup dried chamomile flowers, and 1/4 cup dried rosemary leaves. Store this mixture in an airtight container. Use about 1 cup of this blend per bath. The Epsom salt aids in relaxing muscles, while the herbs contribute their anti-inflammatory and soothing properties.

- Stress Relief Herbal Bath:
  - Ingredients: Dead Sea salts, dried valerian root, dried passion flower, and hops.
  - Recipe: Mix 2 cups of Dead Sea salts with 1/4 cup each of dried valerian root, dried passion flower, and hops. Store the mixture in a jar. Use

1 cup per bath. This combination is excellent for calming the nerves and promoting a sense of deep relaxation.

- Joint Pain Herbal Bath:
  - o Ingredients: Juniper berries, ginger root, and mustard powder.
  - o Recipe: Crush 1/2 cup of dried juniper berries and mix with 1/4 cup of grated ginger root and 1/4 cup of mustard powder. Store the mixture in a dry container. When ready to use, add 1 cup of this blend to your bath. Juniper and ginger are known for their anti-inflammatory properties, while mustard helps in improving circulation.

- Skin Soothing Herbal Bath:
  - o Ingredients: Oatmeal, dried calendula petals, and dried lavender.
  - o Recipe: Grind 1 cup of oatmeal into a fine powder and mix with 1/2 cup of dried calendula petals and 1/2 cup of dried lavender. Store in an airtight container. Add 1 cup of this blend to a warm bath for a soothing and gentle skin-healing experience.

- Detoxifying Herbal Bath:
  - o Ingredients: Bentonite clay, Epsom salt, and peppermint leaves.
  - o Recipe: Mix 1 cup of bentonite clay with 2 cups of Epsom salt and 1/2 cup of dried peppermint leaves. Store the mixture in a jar. Use 1 cup of this blend in your bath for a detoxifying and refreshing experience.

Using Herbal Baths Effectively:

To maximize the benefits of an herbal bath:

- Preparation: Before adding the herbal blend to the bath, consider steeping it in boiling water for 10-15 minutes to create a strong infusion. Strain and add the liquid to the bathwater.
- Hydration: Drink plenty of water before and after the bath to stay hydrated.
- Rest After Bathing: Allow some time to rest after the bath, as the body continues to relax and detoxify.

Herbal baths offer a delightful, natural way to relieve pain and stress, and rejuvenate the body and mind. The recipes provided in this subchapter blend traditional herbal wisdom with modern needs, offering an accessible approach to holistic wellness. By incorporating these soothing baths into your routine, you can enjoy the therapeutic benefits of herbs and the relaxing power of a warm bath, fostering both physical and mental well-being.

CHAPTER 6: MENTAL AND EMOTIONAL WELL-BEING.

In this chapter we delve into the crucial aspect of mental and emotional well-being. This chapter recognizes the intricate connection between the mind, body, and spirit, and focuses on natural and holistic approaches to managing stress, anxiety, depression, mood swings, and sleep disorders. Mental health is as vital as physical health, and this chapter provides insightful guidance on using herbal remedies and relaxation techniques to nurture mental and emotional balance.

The prevalence of mental health issues such as stress, anxiety, and depression has increased significantly in our modern society. Factors contributing to these conditions include the fast-paced lifestyle, constant connectivity, societal pressures, and, in many cases, a disconnection from nature. Herbal remedies offer a gentle yet powerful way to address these challenges. They work not only on the physical symptoms but also on the emotional and spiritual aspects, providing a comprehensive approach to mental health.

Herbal Solutions for Stress and Anxiety:

Stress and anxiety are natural responses to the challenges and demands of life. However, when these responses become chronic, they can lead to a range of physical and mental health issues. Herbal solutions for stress and anxiety include adaptogenic herbs, which help the body adapt to stress, and calming herbs, which soothe the nervous system.

- Adaptogenic Herbs: Adaptogens such as ashwagandha, rhodiola, and ginseng help the body resist stressors, balance stress hormones, and improve overall resilience. These herbs can be taken in various forms, including teas, tinctures, and capsules.
- Calming Herbs: Herbs like chamomile, lavender, and lemon balm are known for their calming effects on the nervous system. They can be particularly helpful in managing anxiety, promoting relaxation, and improving mood.

Natural Treatments for Depression and Mood Swings:

Depression and mood swings can significantly impact one's quality of life. While severe cases require professional medical intervention, mild to moderate symptoms can often be managed with natural treatments. Balancing herbs play a key role in stabilizing mood and improving emotional well-being.

- St. John's Wort: Known for its antidepressant properties, St. John's Wort can be effective in treating mild to moderate depression. It works by increasing the levels of serotonin, a neurotransmitter associated with mood regulation.
- Omega-3 Fatty Acids: Found in fish oil and flaxseeds, omega-3 fatty acids are crucial for brain health and can help alleviate symptoms of depression.
- Saffron: Studies have shown that saffron can be as effective as certain conventional antidepressants in treating mild to moderate depression.

Herbal Sleep Aids and Relaxation Techniques:

Quality sleep is essential for mental and emotional well-being. Insomnia and other sleep disorders can exacerbate stress, anxiety, and depression. Herbal sleep aids, along with relaxation techniques, can significantly improve sleep quality.

- Valerian Root: Valerian is a well-known herbal sleep aid that can help with insomnia. It works by increasing the levels of gamma-aminobutyric acid (GABA), a neurotransmitter that promotes relaxation.
- Lavender: The scent of lavender has a calming effect on the mind and can aid in sleep. Using lavender essential oil in a diffuser or applying it topically can improve sleep quality.
- Relaxation Techniques: Practices such as meditation, deep breathing exercises, and gentle yoga can relax the mind and prepare the body for sleep.

Integrating Herbal Remedies into Daily Life:

Incorporating herbal remedies into one's daily routine can be a transformative practice for mental and emotional health. Whether it's starting the day with an adaptogenic herb blend, taking a calming tea in the evening, or using herbal sleep aids, these natural remedies provide a supportive framework for mental and emotional balance.

- Mindful Consumption: Be mindful of how you consume these herbs. Create a ritual around their intake, whether it's brewing a cup of tea or taking a moment to relax with aromatherapy.

- Consultation with Professionals: Before starting any herbal treatment, especially if you are on medication or have a health condition, consult with a healthcare professional.
- Holistic Approach: Remember that herbs are part of a holistic approach to health. They work best in conjunction with a healthy lifestyle, including a balanced diet, regular exercise, and stress management practices.

In conclusion, Chapter 6 offers a deep insight into managing mental and emotional well-being through herbal remedies and relaxation techniques. By embracing these natural approaches, one can foster a sense of peace, balance, and resilience, crucial for navigating the complexities of modern life. This chapter is a testament to the power of nature in supporting mental and emotional health, offering tools and practices that can be integrated into daily life for lasting well-being.

STRESS AND ANXIETY - HERBAL SOLUTIONS.

In today's fast-paced world, stress and anxiety have become common companions in our daily lives. This subchapter is dedicated to exploring herbal solutions for managing stress and anxiety, with a focus on adaptogenic and calming herbs. These natural remedies offer a holistic approach to soothe the nervous system, balance stress hormones, and promote overall mental well-being.

Stress and anxiety, if left unchecked, can lead to a multitude of health issues, including heart disease, insomnia, and depression. While there are various ways to manage these conditions, including lifestyle changes and therapy, herbal remedies can play a significant role in providing natural relief.

Adaptogenic Herbs for Stress Management:

Adaptogens are a unique class of healing plants that help balance, restore, and protect the body. They have been used for centuries in traditional medicine to help the body resist stressors of all kinds, whether physical, chemical, or biological.

- Ashwagandha: Known as Withania somnifera, ashwagandha is renowned for its stress-relieving properties. It helps to regulate cortisol levels, improving stress response and enhancing overall energy levels.
  - o Ashwagandha Tea Recipe: To make ashwagandha tea, add one teaspoon of ashwagandha powder to a cup of hot water. Let it steep for 10 minutes, then strain and drink. You can sweeten the tea with honey or add a pinch of cinnamon for flavor.

- Rhodiola Rosea: This herb helps improve symptoms of stress, such as fatigue and exhaustion. Rhodiola is known to enhance mental performance and physical stamina.
  - o Rhodiola Tincture Recipe: Fill a jar with dried Rhodiola rosea root and cover it with glycerin

or a non-alcoholic solvent. Let it sit for 4-6 weeks, shaking occasionally. Strain and take 1-2 teaspoons daily.

- Holy Basil (Tulsi): Holy basil is not just a culinary herb; it's a potent adaptogen that helps combat stress and anxiety.
  - Holy Basil Tea Recipe: Steep a handful of fresh holy basil leaves in boiling water for about 5-8 minutes. Strain and enjoy this calming tea, which can be consumed 2-3 times a day.

Calming Herbs for Anxiety Relief:

Calming herbs work by soothing the nervous system, reducing the physical and psychological symptoms of anxiety.

- Chamomile: Chamomile is a gentle, soothing herb, ideal for reducing anxiety and promoting relaxation.
  - Chamomile Infusion Recipe: Add two tablespoons of dried chamomile flowers to a cup of boiling water. Let it steep for about 10 minutes, then strain. Drink this infusion before bedtime to help calm the nerves and promote sleep.

- Lemon Balm: Lemon balm has a natural calming effect and is effective in reducing anxiety and promoting a sense of calm.
  - Lemon Balm Tea Recipe: Brew a tea using dried lemon balm leaves by steeping them in hot

water for about 10 minutes. This can be consumed 2-3 times a day to help ease anxiety.

- Lavender: Lavender is known for its soothing aroma and is widely used in aromatherapy for anxiety relief.
  - o Lavender Oil Aromatherapy: Use a diffuser to disperse lavender essential oil in your living space, or apply diluted lavender oil to the temples and wrists for a calming effect.

Integrating Herbal Remedies into Daily Life:

Incorporating these herbal remedies into daily life involves more than just consumption. It's about creating a holistic lifestyle that supports mental health.

- Mindful Herbal Practices: Engage in a mindful tea-drinking practice, where you focus on the aroma, flavor, and warmth of the tea, allowing it to calm your mind and soothe your nerves.
- Consistent Routines: Establish a routine for taking herbal supplements or teas to ensure consistency, which is key to experiencing their full benefits.
- Balanced Lifestyle: Combine these herbal remedies with a balanced lifestyle that includes regular exercise, a nutritious diet, adequate sleep, and stress-reducing activities like yoga or meditation.

In conclusion, this subchapter provides a detailed guide on using herbal solutions to manage stress and anxiety. These herbs, with their adaptogenic and calming properties, offer a natural pathway to restoring balance and tranquility in our lives. By embracing these herbal practices, alongside a healthy lifestyle, we can navigate life's stresses with greater ease and a more centered state of mind.

DEPRESSION AND MOOD SWINGS - BALANCING HERBS AND NATURAL TREATMENTS.

Depression and mood swings, prevalent in today's society, are complex conditions influenced by a variety of factors, including biological, psychological, and environmental elements. This subchapter delves into natural treatments for depression and mood swings, focusing on balancing herbs that can help stabilize mood and promote emotional well-being. While these treatments can be beneficial, it's important to note that severe depression requires professional medical intervention.

Introduction to Herbal Treatments for Emotional Balance:

Herbs have been used for centuries in various cultures to treat mood disorders and emotional imbalances. These natural treatments often work by influencing the body's stress response, regulating neurotransmitter levels, or alleviating hormonal imbalances, all of which can contribute to mood swings and depression.

- St. John's Wort: St. John's Wort (Hypericum perforatum) is one of the most well-known herbs for treating mild to moderate depression. It is believed to increase the levels of serotonin, norepinephrine, and dopamine in the brain, neurotransmitters linked to mood and emotion.

- o St. John's Wort Tea Recipe: Steep 1-2 teaspoons of dried St. John's Wort in one cup of boiling water for 10 minutes. Strain and drink this tea once or twice daily. Note: St. John's Wort can interact with certain medications, including antidepressants and birth control pills, so it's important to consult a healthcare provider before using this herb.

- Saffron: Studies have shown that saffron (Crocus sativus) can be effective in treating mild to moderate depression. It's thought to work similarly to antidepressants by increasing serotonin levels in the brain.

- o Saffron Tea Recipe: Add a few strands of saffron to a cup of hot water and let it steep for 5 minutes. You can add honey for sweetness. Drink this tea daily for mood enhancement.

- Omega-3 Fatty Acids: While not an herb, omega-3 fatty acids, found in fish oil, flaxseeds, and walnuts, play a crucial role in brain health and can be beneficial in managing depression.

- o Omega-3 Rich Smoothie Recipe: Blend together a handful of spinach, one banana, a tablespoon of flaxseed oil, and a handful of walnuts with your choice of milk. Drink this smoothie daily to incorporate more omega-3s into your diet.

- Ginseng: Ginseng (Panax ginseng) is known for its adaptogenic properties and can be helpful in treating depression and mood swings. It helps in regulating the body's hormonal response to stress and boosts energy levels.
    - Ginseng Infusion Recipe: Add one teaspoon of dried ginseng root to a cup of hot water. Let it steep for 15-20 minutes, then strain. Drink this infusion once daily in the morning.

- Lemon Balm: Lemon balm (Melissa officinalis) is a calming herb that can be beneficial in easing anxiety and mood swings, often associated with depression.
    - Lemon Balm Tea Recipe: Steep 2 teaspoons of dried lemon balm leaves in hot water for 10 minutes. Strain and drink up to three times daily to help calm the nerves and improve mood.

Incorporating Herbs into Daily Life for Emotional Well-being:

Incorporating these herbs into your daily routine can be a comforting and effective way to manage mood swings and symptoms of depression. Here are some additional tips:

- Consistent Use: For these herbs to be effective, they should be used consistently over time. It's important to give them a few weeks to start showing effects.
- Mindful Consumption: Be mindful when consuming these herbs. Pay attention to how your body and mind feel before and after taking them.

- Holistic Approach: Remember that herbs are most effective when combined with a healthy lifestyle. This includes a balanced diet, regular physical activity, adequate sleep, and stress management practices.
- Professional Guidance: Always consult with a healthcare professional before starting any new herbal regimen, especially if you are taking other medications or have existing health conditions.

In conclusion, this subchapter offers a comprehensive look into natural and herbal treatments for depression and mood swings. By understanding and using these herbs mindfully, you can help balance your mood and enhance your emotional well-being. These natural remedies, combined with a healthy lifestyle and professional guidance, can provide a holistic approach to managing mental health challenges.

SLEEP AIDS - HERBAL REMEDIES AND RELAXATION TECHNIQUES FOR IMPROVED SLEEP QUALITY.

Adequate and restful sleep is a cornerstone of good health, impacting our physical, mental, and emotional well-being. This subchapter focuses on natural methods to enhance sleep quality, utilizing herbal sleep aids and relaxation techniques. The remedies and practices discussed here aim to address common sleep issues, such as insomnia and restlessness, offering a holistic approach to achieving restorative sleep.

Introduction to Natural Sleep Aids:

In our modern, fast-paced world, sleep problems have become increasingly common. Factors like stress, screen time, and dietary habits often contribute to sleep disturbances. While there are pharmaceutical options for sleep improvement, natural remedies offer a gentler, side-effect-free alternative. This section delves into herbal solutions and relaxation techniques that promote relaxation and prepare the body and mind for a night of deep, rejuvenating sleep.

Herbal Remedies for Sleep:

Herbs have been used for centuries to aid sleep and treat insomnia. These herbs often contain compounds that relax the nervous system and encourage a state conducive to sleep.

- Valerian Root: Valerian (Valeriana officinalis) is one of the most well-known herbs for sleep. It is believed to increase the levels of gamma-aminobutyric acid (GABA), a neurotransmitter that promotes relaxation.
  - Valerian Root Tea Recipe: Steep 1 teaspoon of dried valerian root in one cup of hot water for 10 minutes. Drink this tea an hour before bedtime. Note: Valerian root has a strong odor, which some may find unpleasant. Adding honey or lemon can help mask the taste.

- Lavender: Lavender is renowned for its calming and sedative properties. It is often used in aromatherapy to reduce stress and improve sleep quality.
  - Lavender Oil Diffusion: Use a diffuser with a few drops of lavender essential oil in your bedroom for about an hour before you go to bed. Alternatively, you can add a few drops of lavender oil to your pillow.

- Chamomile: Chamomile is a gentle, calming herb, effective in promoting relaxation and sleep.
  - Chamomile Tea Recipe: Brew a cup of chamomile tea by steeping 2 tablespoons of dried chamomile flowers in hot water for 10 minutes. Drinking this tea before bed can help soothe the nervous system and prepare the body for sleep.

- Passionflower: Passionflower (Passiflora incarnata) is another herb known for its sleep-inducing properties. It's particularly useful for those with anxiety-related sleep issues.
  - Passionflower Tea Recipe: Infuse 1 teaspoon of dried passionflower in a cup of boiling water for 10 minutes. This tea can be consumed an hour before bedtime to help calm the mind.

- Lemon Balm: Lemon balm has a soothing effect and can be used to ease stress and anxiety, promoting better sleep.
  - Lemon Balm and Mint Tea: Mix equal parts of dried lemon balm and mint. Steep in hot water for about 10 minutes, strain, and enjoy this calming tea in the evening.

Relaxation Techniques for Improved Sleep:

In addition to herbal remedies, various relaxation techniques can be employed to improve sleep quality.

- Mindful Meditation: Practice mindfulness meditation for 10-15 minutes before bed. Focus on your breath and allow thoughts to pass without engagement, which can help quiet the mind.

- Progressive Muscle Relaxation: Starting at your toes and moving up to your head, tense each muscle group for a few seconds and then release. This technique helps reduce physical tension and promote relaxation.

- Deep Breathing Exercises: Engage in deep, slow breathing to activate the body's relaxation response. Try the 4-7-8 breathing technique, where you inhale for 4 seconds, hold the breath for 7 seconds, and exhale for 8 seconds.

- Yoga for Sleep: Gentle yoga poses, particularly those that focus on relaxation, can be done before bed to prepare the body for sleep. Poses like Child's Pose, Legs Up the Wall, and Corpse Pose are especially beneficial.

- Creating a Sleep-Inducing Environment: Ensure your bedroom is conducive to sleep; cool, dark, and quiet.

Consider using blackout curtains, earplugs, or white noise machines if needed.

In conclusion, this subchapter offers a comprehensive guide on using herbal remedies and relaxation techniques to improve sleep quality. By integrating these natural approaches into your nightly routine, you can encourage a more restful and restorative sleep, essential for overall health and well-being. These practices, when combined with a healthy lifestyle, can significantly enhance your sleep quality, contributing to improved mental, emotional, and physical health.

CHAPTER 7: WOMEN'S AND MEN'S HEALTH.

This Chapter is a comprehensive guide dedicated to addressing the unique health needs and challenges faced by women and men. This chapter explores a range of natural and herbal remedies tailored to support specific health concerns related to women's menstrual discomfort and menopause symptoms, as well as men's prostate health and hormonal balance. Additionally, it delves into the broader topic of hormonal balance, offering insight into herbs and dietary advice beneficial for both genders.

Understanding and addressing the distinct health needs of women and men is crucial for overall well-being. Women often face health challenges related to their reproductive system, such as menstrual discomfort and menopause, while men may encounter issues related to prostate health and hormonal imbalances. This chapter aims to provide natural solutions and preventative measures to support and improve health specific to each gender.

Herbal Remedies for Women's Health:

Women's health, particularly concerning reproductive health, can be complex and multifaceted. Herbal remedies can be particularly effective in addressing issues such as menstrual discomfort, premenstrual syndrome (PMS), and symptoms associated with menopause. These remedies often focus on regulating hormones, alleviating pain, and providing emotional and physical balance.

- Menstrual Discomfort: Various herbs can help alleviate menstrual cramps and discomfort. Herbs like ginger, cramp bark, and raspberry leaf are known for their ability to relieve menstrual pain and regulate menstrual cycles.
- Menopause Symptoms: Menopause can bring a range of symptoms, from hot flashes to mood swings. Herbs like black cohosh, red clover, and sage have been traditionally used to ease these symptoms. They work by providing phytoestrogens and supporting hormonal balance.

Natural Treatments for Men's Health:

Men's health issues, particularly as they age, often revolve around prostate health and hormonal balance. Natural treatments and preventive measures can play a significant role in maintaining prostate health and ensuring hormonal equilibrium.

- Prostate Health: Herbs like saw palmetto and pygeum are popular for supporting prostate health. They are known to help with benign prostatic hyperplasia (BPH) symptoms and promote overall prostate well-being.
- Hormonal Balance in Men: Hormonal balance is crucial for men's health, affecting everything from mood to muscle strength. Herbs such as ashwagandha and fenugreek can help in maintaining this balance, improving energy levels, and enhancing overall vitality.

Maintaining Hormonal Balance:

Hormonal balance is not exclusive to women or men; it is a vital aspect of health for both. An imbalance can lead to a variety of health issues, from stress and fatigue to more serious chronic conditions. This section of the chapter addresses how both women and men can maintain hormonal balance through herbs and diet.

- Adaptogenic Herbs: Adaptogens like Rhodiola and Holy Basil can help the body adapt to stress, a major factor in hormonal imbalance. These herbs support the adrenal glands and help regulate the production of cortisol, a stress hormone.
- Diet and Lifestyle: A diet rich in whole foods, healthy fats, and antioxidants supports hormonal health. Foods like avocados, nuts, seeds, and leafy greens are particularly beneficial. Regular exercise, adequate sleep, and stress reduction techniques are also crucial for hormonal balance.

In conclusion, Chapter 7 offers an in-depth exploration of women's and men's health issues and how they can be effectively addressed through natural remedies and lifestyle adjustments. This chapter not only provides practical guidance on specific health concerns but also emphasizes the importance of a holistic approach to maintaining hormonal balance and overall well-being. By understanding and addressing the unique health needs of each gender, this chapter serves as a valuable resource for anyone seeking to enhance their health naturally and harmoniously.

WOMEN'S HEALTH - HERBAL REMEDIES FOR MENSTRUAL DISCOMFORT AND MENOPAUSE SYMPTOMS.

Women's health, particularly concerning menstrual discomfort and menopause symptoms, involves a complex interplay of hormones and physiological changes. In this subchapter, we explore in-depth herbal remedies that can provide relief from menstrual pain and menopause-related issues. These natural treatments are aimed at not just alleviating symptoms but also at nurturing the overall well-being of women during these challenging phases of their lives.

Introduction to Herbal Care for Women's Health:

The use of herbs for women's health is a time-honored tradition, rooted in ancient practices. Herbs can offer significant relief from menstrual cramps, mood swings, hot flashes, and other symptoms associated with menstrual cycles and menopause. These remedies work by balancing hormones, reducing inflammation, and providing calming effects.

Herbal Remedies for Menstrual Discomfort:

Menstrual discomfort, including cramps and mood swings, is a common issue faced by many women during their menstrual cycle. Herbs can play a key role in managing these symptoms.

- Raspberry Leaf Tea for Cramp Relief: Raspberry leaf is a uterine tonic that can help in strengthening uterine muscles and relieving menstrual cramps.
  - Recipe: Steep 2 tablespoons of dried raspberry leaves in a cup of boiling water for about 15 minutes. Strain and drink this tea 1-2 times a day, starting a few days before the onset of menstruation.

- Chamomile Tea for Relaxation: Chamomile has anti-inflammatory properties that can help soothe menstrual cramps and also aids in relaxation.
  - Recipe: Infuse 2 teaspoons of dried chamomile flowers in hot water for 10 minutes. Drinking this tea during menstruation can provide pain relief and calmness.

- Ginger Root for Inflammation: Ginger is effective in reducing menstrual pain and inflammation.
  - Recipe: Slice fresh ginger root and simmer in water for 15 minutes. Strain and add honey for flavor. Consume this warm ginger tea two to three times a day during periods.

Herbal Approaches to Menopause Symptoms:

Menopause brings a range of symptoms from hot flashes to sleep disturbances. Herbal remedies can be particularly helpful in managing these symptoms.

- Black Cohosh for Hot Flashes: Black cohosh is widely used for relieving menopause symptoms, particularly hot flashes and night sweats.
    o Recipe: Black cohosh is best taken in capsule or tincture form as per the recommended dosage on the product label. Ensure to consult with a healthcare provider before starting any new supplement.

- Sage Tea for Excessive Sweating: Sage helps in reducing night sweats and hot flashes associated with menopause.
    o Recipe: Steep 1 teaspoon of dried sage leaves in boiling water for about 10 minutes. Strain and drink this tea once daily.

- Red Clover for Hormonal Balance: Red clover contains isoflavones, plant-based chemicals that mimic estrogen in the body.
    o Recipe: Add 1-2 teaspoons of dried red clover flowers to a cup of hot water. Steep for 15 minutes, strain, and drink 1-2 cups daily.

Supporting Women's Health with Lifestyle and Diet:

In addition to herbal remedies, supporting women's health during menstruation and menopause also involves dietary and lifestyle considerations.

- Nutrition for Hormonal Balance: Include foods rich in phytoestrogens, such as flaxseeds and soy products, as well as calcium-rich foods like dairy or fortified plant milks, and leafy greens.

- Regular Exercise: Engage in regular physical activity to help alleviate menstrual pain and menopause symptoms. Activities like yoga, walking, and swimming can be particularly beneficial.
- Stress Management: Practices such as meditation, deep breathing exercises, and mindfulness can help manage stress, which is often a contributing factor to menstrual and menopausal discomfort.

In conclusion, this subchapter offers a holistic approach to managing women's health issues related to menstruation and menopause. By understanding and utilizing these herbal remedies, along with supportive lifestyle and dietary practices, women can find relief from discomfort and improve their overall well-being. It's important to remember that every woman's body is different, and what works for one may not work for another. Consulting with a healthcare provider before starting any new treatment is always advised.

MEN'S HEALTH - FOCUSING ON PROSTATE HEALTH AND HORMONAL BALANCE

Men's health, particularly regarding prostate health and hormonal balance, is an essential aspect of overall well-being that often gets overlooked. This subchapter is dedicated to addressing these specific areas with natural treatments and herbal remedies. The focus is not only on alleviating symptoms associated with prostate issues and hormonal imbalances but also on promoting long-term health and prevention strategies.

Introduction to Men's Health Concerns:

As men age, they often face unique health challenges, such as prostate enlargement or benign prostatic hyperplasia (BPH), and issues related to hormonal imbalances, including reduced testosterone levels. These conditions can significantly impact life quality, making it crucial to address them proactively. Herbal remedies and natural treatments can play a significant role in supporting men's health, offering a holistic approach to maintaining wellbeing.

Herbal Treatments for Prostate Health:

The prostate, a small gland in men, tends to enlarge with age, leading to discomfort and health issues like BPH. Several herbs have been shown to support prostate health and alleviate symptoms.

- Saw Palmetto Berry Extract: Saw palmetto is perhaps the most well-known herb for prostate health. It helps in reducing the symptoms of BPH and maintaining prostate function.
  - Recipe for Saw Palmetto Berry Tea: Steep 1 teaspoon of dried saw palmetto berries in hot water for about 10 minutes. Strain and drink this tea daily. Saw palmetto is also available in capsule and tincture form, which can be taken as directed on the product label.

- Nettle Root: Nettle root is another herb that benefits prostate health, particularly in combination with saw palmetto.
  - o Nettle Root Tea Recipe: Add 1 tablespoon of dried nettle root to a cup of boiling water. Let it steep for about 10 minutes, then strain and drink. Consuming this tea once or twice a day can support prostate health.

- Pygeum: Derived from the bark of the African plum tree, pygeum is traditionally used for treating BPH symptoms.
  - o Pygeum Supplement: Pygeum is typically taken in capsule form. Follow the dosage instructions provided on the supplement bottle.

Natural Approaches for Hormonal Balance in Men:

Maintaining hormonal balance, particularly testosterone levels, is vital for men's health. Certain herbs and foods can naturally support hormonal balance.

- Ashwagandha for Stress and Testosterone Levels: Ashwagandha is known for its adaptogenic properties, helping the body manage stress and potentially supporting healthy testosterone levels.
  - o Ashwagandha Infusion: Mix a teaspoon of ashwagandha powder in a cup of hot water or milk. Add honey for taste and consume daily.

- Fenugreek for Hormonal Support: Fenugreek seeds are believed to support testosterone levels and improve overall health.
  - Fenugreek Seed Tea: Soak fenugreek seeds overnight in water. Boil this water with seeds the next morning for about 5 minutes, then strain and drink.

- Ginger Root for Antioxidant Support: Ginger has antioxidant properties and may have a positive effect on testosterone levels.
  - Ginger Root Tea: Slice fresh ginger root and simmer in water for about 15 minutes. Strain and add a bit of honey or lemon. Drink this tea daily for its health benefits.

Lifestyle and Dietary Tips for Men's Health:

In addition to herbal remedies, certain lifestyle and dietary changes can significantly benefit prostate health and hormonal balance.

- Regular Exercise: Engaging in regular physical activity can help maintain a healthy weight, reduce stress, and support hormonal balance.
- Healthy Diet: Incorporating foods rich in zinc (like oysters, beef, and pumpkin seeds), omega-3 fatty acids (such as salmon and walnuts), and antioxidants (found in fruits and vegetables) can support prostate health and hormonal balance.

- Hydration and Moderation: Staying well-hydrated and moderating the intake of caffeine and alcohol can also be beneficial for prostate health.
- Stress Management: Practices like meditation, yoga, and deep breathing exercises can help manage stress, which is crucial for hormonal balance.

In conclusion, this subchapter provides in-depth insights into natural treatments and lifestyle approaches for improving men's health, focusing on prostate health and hormonal balance. By incorporating these herbal remedies and lifestyle adjustments, men can proactively manage their health, leading to improved wellbeing and quality of life. It's important to remember that while these natural approaches can be highly effective, they should complement regular medical check-ups and consultations with healthcare professionals.

HORMONAL BALANCE - HERBS AND DIETARY STRATEGIES

Maintaining hormonal balance is essential for overall health and well-being for both women and men. Hormones, acting as the body's chemical messengers, play a critical role in regulating various physiological processes. Imbalances can lead to a myriad of health issues, ranging from mood swings and weight gain to more serious conditions like infertility and metabolic disorders. This subchapter is dedicated to exploring herbs and dietary advice aimed at maintaining hormonal balance, providing practical, natural solutions for achieving and sustaining this balance.

Introduction to Hormonal Balance:

Hormonal balance is not just about addressing specific health issues but is integral to the optimal functioning of the entire body. Both excess and deficiency of hormones can cause health problems. For instance, excess cortisol can lead to stress and weight gain, while insufficient thyroid hormones can result in fatigue and depression. The natural approaches discussed here are aimed at stabilizing hormone levels, thus supporting the body's natural rhythm and overall health.

Herbal Remedies for Hormonal Balance:

Certain herbs have been recognized for their ability to regulate hormones and support endocrine system health. These herbal remedies can be incorporated into daily routines to help maintain hormonal balance.

- Ashwagandha for Stress Hormones: Ashwagandha is an adaptogen, meaning it helps the body adapt to stress. It can be particularly effective in balancing cortisol levels.
  - Ashwagandha Milk Recipe: Mix half a teaspoon of ashwagandha powder into a cup of warm milk. Add a teaspoon of honey for sweetness and drink before bedtime. This can help regulate stress hormones and improve sleep quality.

- Maca Root for Reproductive Hormones: Maca root is known for its ability to enhance fertility and balance sex hormones in both men and women.
  - Maca Smoothie Recipe: Blend a teaspoon of maca powder with your favorite fruits, a handful of spinach, and a cup of almond milk. This nutritious smoothie can be consumed daily.

- Chaste Tree Berry (Vitex) for Female Hormonal Balance: Chaste tree berry is particularly beneficial for women, helping to regulate menstrual cycles and alleviate symptoms of PMS.
  - Chaste Tree Berry Tea: Steep one teaspoon of dried chaste tree berries in hot water for 10 minutes. Strain and drink once daily in the morning.

- Saw Palmetto for Male Hormonal Health: Saw palmetto is beneficial for prostate health and balancing testosterone levels in men.
  - Saw Palmetto Capsule: Saw palmetto is best taken in capsule form, as per the dosage instructions on the product label.

Dietary Advice for Hormonal Health:

Diet plays a crucial role in maintaining hormonal balance. Certain foods can naturally support hormonal health by providing essential nutrients, supporting detoxification, and stabilizing blood sugar levels.

- Omega-3 Fatty Acids: Foods rich in omega-3 fatty acids, like fatty fish, flaxseeds, and walnuts, are vital for hormonal balance, particularly in reducing inflammation.

- Fiber-Rich Foods: High-fiber foods, such as fruits, vegetables, and whole grains, help in the digestion and excretion of excess hormones.

- Cruciferous Vegetables: Vegetables like broccoli, cauliflower, and Brussels sprouts contain indole-3-carbinol, which can help in balancing estrogen levels.
- Probiotic Foods: Fermented foods like yogurt, kefir, and sauerkraut support gut health, which is crucial for hormone metabolism.

- Blood Sugar Balancing Foods: Maintaining stable blood sugar levels is vital for hormonal health. Incorporate foods with a low glycemic index, such as whole grains and legumes, and pair carbohydrates with proteins or healthy fats.

Lifestyle Factors Influencing Hormonal Balance:

In addition to herbs and diet, certain lifestyle factors are important in maintaining hormonal balance.

- Regular Exercise: Regular physical activity can help balance hormones by reducing insulin levels and increasing insulin sensitivity.

- Adequate Sleep: Quality sleep is essential for hormonal balance, particularly for regulating cortisol and insulin.
- Stress Management: Chronic stress can lead to hormonal imbalances, particularly in cortisol and adrenaline levels. Practices such as yoga, meditation, and mindfulness can help manage stress.
- Avoiding Endocrine Disruptors: Be mindful of endocrine disruptors found in certain plastics, personal care products, and pesticides. Opting for natural and organic products can reduce exposure to these harmful chemicals.

In conclusion, this subchapter provides a comprehensive approach to maintaining hormonal balance through natural herbs and dietary strategies. By integrating these practices into daily life, along with healthy lifestyle choices, both women and men can support their hormonal health, leading to improved physical and mental well-being. It's important to approach hormonal balance as a holistic process, encompassing diet, lifestyle, and natural remedies, to achieve optimal health.

CHAPTER 8: HERBAL FIRST AID KIT.

In this chapter we introduce the concept of an herbal first aid kit, a natural and effective complement to traditional first aid methods. This chapter is a guide to creating and using a herbal first aid kit for various common health concerns, including minor injuries, headaches, migraines, and everyday ailments. The focus is on quick, accessible, and practical herbal treatments that can be prepared and used at home or on the go.

The Essence of an Herbal First Aid Kit:

The idea of a herbal first aid kit stems from the understanding that nature offers us a plethora of plants with medicinal properties, capable of providing immediate relief for an array of minor health issues. Unlike conventional medicine, herbal remedies often come with fewer side effects and can be a holistic alternative or supplement to over-the-counter medications. This chapter aims to educate on how to effectively harness the power of these herbs for first aid purposes.

Preparing Your Herbal First Aid Kit:

A well-stocked herbal first aid kit includes a variety of herbs and natural substances that are versatile and effective for treating common ailments. The key is to select herbs based on their medicinal properties and the types of emergencies they can address.

- Essential Herbs and Natural Substances: Your kit should include herbs like calendula (for skin healing), lavender (for burns and stress relief), chamomile (for soothing and anti-inflammatory properties), peppermint (for digestive issues), and Echinacea (for immune support).
- Forms of Herbs: Herbs can be kept in various forms, such as dried herbs, tinctures, essential oils, and salves. Each form has its own method of application and shelf life.
- Storage and Accessibility: Store your herbal first aid kit in a cool, dry place, and ensure it's easily accessible. A portable version can be useful for travel.

Application of Herbal First Aid:

The practical application of these herbs depends on the nature of the ailment.

- Cuts and Wounds: Herbs like calendula and yarrow can be used for their antiseptic and healing properties. A salve or poultice made from these herbs can be applied to clean cuts to promote healing.

- Burns: Aloe vera and lavender essential oil are excellent for treating minor burns. They provide soothing relief and aid in skin repair.

- Bites and Stings: Plantain leaves and tea tree oil can be used to relieve the pain and itching from insect bites and stings.

In-Depth Treatments in the Herbal First Aid Kit:

The effectiveness of an herbal first aid kit lies in knowing how to use each component.

- Herbal Salves: Salves made from comfrey, calendula, or plantain are great for treating minor skin irritations, cuts, and burns. They create a protective barrier and support the skin's natural healing process.

- Herbal Teas and Tinctures: For internal issues like indigestion or nausea, herbal teas or tinctures can be effective. Peppermint and ginger are excellent choices for digestive discomfort.

- Essential Oils: Oils like lavender and peppermint are versatile and can be used for headaches, stress relief, and respiratory issues.

In conclusion, this chapter empowers readers with the knowledge and tools to address common health concerns using natural remedies. It highlights the importance of understanding each herb's properties and how to apply them effectively in various situations. By integrating these herbal solutions into your first aid practices, you can manage minor health issues more naturally and holistically. Remember, while herbal remedies are beneficial for minor issues, serious injuries and health concerns should always be addressed by a healthcare professional.

MINOR INJURIES - QUICK HERBAL TREATMENTS FOR CUTS, BURNS, AND BITES.

In the realm of natural healing, addressing minor injuries such as cuts, burns, and insect bites with herbal remedies can be both effective and satisfying. This subchapter delves into practical, easy-to-prepare herbal treatments that can be a cornerstone of any home first aid kit. These natural remedies offer a gentle yet potent alternative to conventional treatments, harnessing the healing powers of herbs to provide relief and promote healing.

Introduction to Herbal Care for Minor Injuries:

Minor injuries, while generally not life-threatening, require proper care to prevent infection and promote healing. Herbs, with their diverse medicinal properties, can play a crucial role in this process. They offer natural antiseptic, anti-inflammatory, and analgesic properties, making them ideal for treating minor wounds, burns, and bites. This section presents a range of herbal treatments, from poultices and salves to infusions and washes, each tailored to treat specific types of minor injuries.

Herbal Remedies for Cuts and Scrapes:

Cuts and scrapes are common injuries that can be effectively treated with herbs known for their antiseptic and healing properties.

- Calendula Wash for Cuts: Calendula is renowned for its wound-healing properties. It helps in reducing inflammation and promoting tissue repair.
  - Recipe: Brew a strong infusion of calendula flowers by steeping 2 tablespoons of dried flowers in a cup of boiling water for about 15 minutes. Once cooled, use this infusion to gently clean the cut or scrape.

-

- Comfrey Poultice for Rapid Healing: Comfrey is known for its ability to speed up the healing process of cuts and bruises.
  - Recipe: Crush fresh comfrey leaves to create a poultice. Apply this directly to the cut and secure with a clean bandage. Change the poultice every few hours.

-

- Yarrow Powder to Stop Bleeding: Yarrow is effective in stopping bleeding and can be used on fresh cuts.
  - Recipe: Grind dried yarrow leaves and flowers into a fine powder. Sprinkle this powder directly onto the cut to help stop bleeding and begin the healing process.

Natural Treatments for Burns:

Burns, ranging from minor to severe, require immediate care. Herbs can provide soothing relief and aid in skin repair.

- Aloe Vera Gel for Immediate Relief: Aloe vera is widely used for treating minor burns due to its soothing and cooling properties.
    - Recipe: Slice open an aloe vera leaf and apply the fresh gel directly to the burn. Reapply as needed for relief.

- Lavender Oil for Burn Care: Lavender essential oil is beneficial for minor burns as it provides pain relief and supports healing.
    - Recipe: Dilute a few drops of lavender essential oil in a carrier oil like coconut oil and apply gently to the burn area.

Herbal Solutions for Bites and Stings:

Insect bites and stings can be itchy and painful but respond well to certain herbs known for their anti-inflammatory and soothing properties.

- Plantain Leaf Poultice for Bites: Plantain leaves are effective in relieving the itchiness and discomfort of insect bites.
    - Recipe: Chew or crush fresh plantain leaves to release their juice. Apply this directly to the bite or sting for relief.

- Tea Tree Oil for Antiseptic Action: Tea tree oil is a natural antiseptic and can be used to treat insect bites.

o   Recipe: Dilute tea tree oil with a carrier oil and apply to the bite to reduce inflammation and prevent infection.

Incorporating Herbal Remedies into First Aid Practices:

Using these herbal remedies requires some basic knowledge and preparation. Keep these points in mind:

- Freshness and Quality: Use fresh or well-preserved herbs to ensure the efficacy of the remedies.
- Patch Test: Especially when using essential oils or new herbs, do a patch test to rule out any allergic reactions.
- Hygiene: Ensure cleanliness while preparing and applying these remedies to avoid infection.
- Know When to Seek Professional Help: While effective for minor injuries, professional medical care is essential for serious wounds, deep burns, or if there are signs of infection.

In conclusion, this subchapter provides a detailed guide on preparing and using herbal treatments for minor injuries. By harnessing the natural healing properties of herbs, you can effectively address common injuries like cuts, burns, and bites in a safe, natural, and effective way. As with all home remedies, these treatments are intended for minor injuries, and more serious conditions should be evaluated and treated by healthcare professionals.

HEADACHES AND MIGRAINES - HERBAL REMEDIES FOR RELIEF

Headaches and migraines are common ailments affecting a large portion of the population. They can range from mild discomfort to debilitating pain and can significantly impact daily life. This subchapter explores various herbal remedies for both preventing and treating headaches and migraines. By understanding and utilizing the therapeutic properties of specific herbs, individuals can find natural relief and potentially reduce the frequency and intensity of these episodes.

Introduction to Herbal Treatment of Headaches and Migraines:

Headaches and migraines can have various triggers, including stress, dehydration, hormonal changes, and dietary factors. While over-the-counter medications are commonly used for relief, herbal remedies offer an effective and natural alternative with fewer side effects. These remedies work by addressing the underlying causes of headaches, such as tension, inflammation, or vascular changes.

Preventative Herbal Strategies for Headaches and Migraines:

Prevention is a key strategy in managing headaches and migraines. Certain herbs can be used regularly to reduce the likelihood of occurrences.

- Feverfew for Migraine Prevention: Feverfew is a well-known herb for preventing migraines. It reduces inflammation, which is often a contributing factor in migraine headaches.
  - Feverfew Tea Recipe: Steep 1 teaspoon of dried feverfew leaves in a cup of hot water for 10 minutes. Strain and drink this tea daily as a preventive measure.

- Butterbur for Reducing Frequency of Migraines: Butterbur has been shown to reduce the frequency of migraine attacks.
  - Butterbur Capsule Regimen: Butterbur is best taken in capsule form. Choose a product that is PA (pyrrolizidine alkaloids) free and follow the dosage instructions on the bottle.

- Magnesium-Rich Herbal Infusions: Magnesium is known to help prevent migraines. Herbs like nettle and oat straw are high in magnesium.
  - Magnesium-Rich Herbal Infusion: Combine equal parts of dried nettle and oat straw. Steep a handful in hot water for 4 hours or overnight. Strain and drink this infusion daily.

Acute Herbal Remedies for Headaches:

When a headache strikes, quick relief is key. Certain herbs can be used to alleviate pain and relax tense muscles.

- Peppermint Oil for Tension Headaches: Peppermint oil is effective in relieving tension headaches when applied topically.
    - Peppermint Oil Application: Dilute peppermint essential oil with a carrier oil and gently massage onto the temples and back of the neck. The cooling effect of peppermint can provide immediate relief.

- Ginger for Inflammation and Nausea: Ginger is an anti-inflammatory herb that can help reduce the pain of headaches and is particularly useful for migraines with nausea.
    - Ginger Tea Recipe: Simmer slices of fresh ginger root in water for 15 minutes. Strain, add honey for taste, and drink at the onset of headache symptoms.

- Lavender Oil for Relaxation: Lavender oil has calming properties that can be beneficial during a headache or migraine.
    - Lavender Oil Aromatherapy: Use lavender oil in a diffuser or apply diluted oil to the temples. The relaxing aroma can help ease headache pain.

Lifestyle and Dietary Considerations for Headache and Migraine Sufferers:

In conjunction with herbal remedies, certain lifestyle and dietary changes can help manage headaches and migraines.

- Hydration: Dehydration can be a trigger for headaches. Ensure adequate water intake throughout the day.
- Stress Management: Since stress is a common trigger for headaches, incorporating stress-reduction techniques such as yoga, meditation, and deep breathing exercises can be beneficial.
- Regular Exercise: Physical activity can reduce the frequency and severity of headaches by improving overall health and reducing stress.
- Dietary Adjustments: Identify and avoid foods that trigger headaches. Common culprits include caffeine, alcohol, aged cheeses, and processed foods.

In conclusion, this subchapter provides a comprehensive overview of using herbal remedies for the prevention and treatment of headaches and migraines. By integrating these natural treatments with lifestyle and dietary adjustments, individuals can achieve greater control over their headache and migraine symptoms, leading to improved quality of life. Remember, while herbal remedies can be highly effective, they should be used in consultation with a healthcare provider, especially for individuals with frequent or severe headaches.

COMMON AILMENTS - HERBAL RECIPES FOR EVERYDAY RELIEF

Everyday ailments like indigestion, fatigue, and insomnia, though not usually severe, can significantly affect our daily lives and overall well-being. In this subchapter, we delve into the world of herbal remedies, focusing on practical and effective solutions for these common issues. Using herbs for these conditions not only addresses the symptoms but often targets the root causes, offering a holistic approach to health and wellness.

Introduction to Herbal Solutions for Everyday Ailments:

Herbal remedies have been used for centuries to treat everyday ailments. These natural solutions are often gentler on the body than conventional medications and can be used as part of an ongoing wellness routine. This section explores various herbal recipes that can be easily prepared and used at home to alleviate common issues like indigestion, fatigue, and insomnia.

Herbal Remedies for Indigestion:

Indigestion, a common digestive issue, can be caused by factors like overeating, stress, or certain foods. Herbal remedies can aid digestion, relieve discomfort, and promote gut health.

- Peppermint Tea for Digestive Relief: Peppermint has antispasmodic properties, making it effective in soothing stomach cramps and relieving gas.
  - Recipe: Steep 1-2 teaspoons of dried peppermint leaves in a cup of boiling water for 10 minutes. Drink this tea after meals to aid digestion and relieve symptoms of indigestion.

- Ginger and Honey Digestive Tonic: Ginger stimulates digestion and has a calming effect on the digestive system.
  - Recipe: Simmer slices of fresh ginger in water for 15 minutes. Strain and add a teaspoon of honey to the warm ginger tea. Drink as needed to alleviate indigestion.

- Fennel Seed Infusion for Bloating: Fennel seeds are known for their ability to reduce bloating and gas.
  - Recipe: Crush a teaspoon of fennel seeds and steep them in boiling water for 10 minutes. Strain and drink this infusion after meals to help with bloating.

Herbal Solutions for Fatigue:

Fatigue can be due to various factors, including stress, poor sleep, and nutritional deficiencies. Certain herbs can help boost energy levels and improve overall vitality.

- Ginseng for Energy Boost: Ginseng is a well-known adaptogen that helps increase energy levels and improve stamina.
  - Recipe: Ginseng is best taken in tincture or capsule form. Follow the recommended dosage on the product label for the best results.

- Ashwagandha for Stress-Related Fatigue: Ashwagandha helps the body adapt to stress and can be beneficial in combating stress-related fatigue.
  - Recipe: Mix half a teaspoon of ashwagandha powder in a glass of warm milk. Drink this mixture once daily to help rejuvenate the body.

- Green Tea and Lemon for Sustained Energy: Green tea provides a gentle energy boost without the jitters often associated with coffee.
  - Recipe: Brew green tea and add a slice of lemon. The combination of caffeine and vitamin C can help improve energy levels.

Natural Remedies for Insomnia:

Insomnia, the inability to fall or stay asleep, can significantly impact health and quality of life. Herbal remedies can be a natural way to promote restful sleep.

- Valerian Root Tea for Deep Sleep: Valerian root is a natural sedative and can help improve sleep quality.
  - Recipe: Steep 1 teaspoon of dried valerian root in a cup of hot water for 10 minutes. Drink this tea 30 minutes before bedtime to aid sleep.

- Lavender and Chamomile Sleepy-Time Tea: Lavender and chamomile are both known for their calming and relaxing properties.
  - Recipe: Mix equal parts of dried lavender and chamomile. Steep a tablespoon of this blend in hot water for 10 minutes. Drink this tea before bedtime to encourage relaxation and sleep.

- Lemon Balm for a Calm Mind: Lemon balm can help reduce anxiety and promote a sense of calm, making it easier to fall asleep.

o   Recipe: Steep dried lemon balm leaves in boiling water for 10 minutes. Drinking this tea in the evening can help prepare the mind for sleep.

Incorporating Herbal Remedies into Daily Life:

Integrating these herbal remedies into your daily routine can be a simple yet effective way to manage common ailments.

- Consistency is Key: Regular use of these remedies can provide the best results, especially for chronic issues like indigestion and insomnia.
- Quality of Herbs: Always use high-quality, organic herbs to ensure the efficacy of the remedies.
- Listen to Your Body: Pay attention to how your body responds to these remedies and adjust accordingly. What works for one person may not work for another.

In conclusion, this subchapter offers a comprehensive guide to using herbal remedies for treating everyday ailments such as indigestion, fatigue, and insomnia. By understanding the properties of different herbs and how to use them effectively, you can address these common issues naturally and safely. As with any treatment, it's important to consider individual health conditions and consult with a healthcare provider when necessary. These natural solutions, when integrated into a holistic health approach, can greatly enhance your overall well-being.

CHAPTER 9: SEASONAL HERBAL REMEDIES

This chapter is dedicated to exploring how the changing seasons affect our health and how we can use herbal remedies to adapt and thrive throughout the year. From the cold grips of winter to the warm embrace of summer, each season brings its unique challenges and opportunities for natural wellness. Here, we delve into the world of seasonal herbalism, offering insights and practical remedies to align our health practices with the rhythms of nature.

The Essence of Seasonal Herbalism:

Seasonal herbalism is based on the understanding that our bodies are inextricably linked to the natural world. As the seasons change, so do our bodies' needs. Winter, for example, might call for immune-boosting herbs to ward off colds and flu, while summer may require remedies for sunburn or insect bites. By tuning into these seasonal needs and using herbs that are naturally available or particularly effective at certain times of the year, we can enhance our health and well-being in a harmonious and sustainable way.

Understanding the Body's Seasonal Needs:

Our bodies respond to the changes in light, temperature, and environmental factors that each season brings. In winter, the body conserves energy and often requires support for the immune system. Spring brings renewal and often a need for cleansing and rejuvenation. Summer, with its abundance of light and warmth, can sometimes lead to overexposure-related issues like sunburn. Autumn is a time of preparation for the colder months, focusing on nourishing and strengthening the body.

Immunity Boosters for Cold and Flu Season:

One of the key focuses of seasonal herbal remedies is boosting immunity during the colder months. As the body becomes more susceptible to colds and flu, certain herbs can be particularly beneficial.

- Echinacea for Immune Support: Echinacea is a go-to herb for enhancing the immune system and is particularly effective when taken at the onset of cold or flu symptoms.

- Elderberry for Antiviral Protection: Elderberry has antiviral properties, making it useful in preventing and treating colds and flu.

- Ginger and Turmeric for Inflammation: Both ginger and turmeric have anti-inflammatory properties and can help alleviate symptoms of colds, such as sore throats and congestion.

Herbal Treatments for Summer Issues:

Summer brings its own set of challenges, including sunburn, insect bites, and overheating. Certain herbs can provide relief and protection during the warmer months.

- Aloe Vera for Sunburn: Aloe vera is well-known for its soothing properties and is excellent for treating sunburn.

- Calendula for Skin Irritation: Calendula is beneficial for various skin irritations that can occur during summer, including insect bites and rashes.

- Peppermint for Cooling: Peppermint has a natural cooling effect and can be used in foot baths or as a diluted essential oil for a refreshing, cooling sensation.

Adapting Herbal Remedies According to Seasonal Changes:

Adapting to the seasons doesn't just involve using different herbs; it also includes changing our approach to how we use them. For instance, teas and infusions might be more appropriate in winter, while tinctures or fresh herbal juices might be preferable in summer.

In conclusion, Chapter 9 offers an enlightening journey through the seasons with herbal remedies tailored for each period's unique needs. This chapter empowers readers with the knowledge to use nature's offerings wisely and effectively, aligning their health practices with the ebb and flow of the seasons. Embracing seasonal herbalism not only enhances our connection to the natural world but also allows us to live in greater harmony with our own bodies' rhythms and needs. By understanding and implementing these seasonal herbal strategies, we open the door to a more holistic and attuned way of living and healing.

IMMUNITY BOOSTERS - HERBAL REMEDIES FOR COLD AND FLU SEASON.

In the colder months, our immune systems often require extra support to guard against common ailments like colds and flu. This subchapter delves into the world of herbal remedies, focusing on natural ways to bolster immunity during these vulnerable times. These remedies, steeped in traditional wisdom and backed by modern research, offer effective and natural alternatives to enhance our body's defenses.

Introduction to Immunity-Boosting Herbal Remedies:

Boosting immunity is not just about fighting off an imminent cold or flu; it's about nurturing the body's inherent ability to defend itself. Herbal remedies can be powerful allies in this endeavor, offering a range of benefits from antiviral properties to immune system enhancement. Here, we explore a variety of herbs known for their immune-boosting capabilities and provide practical recipes to incorporate them into your daily routine.

Key Herbs for Immune Support:

Several herbs stand out for their ability to strengthen the immune system and help the body resist infections.

- Echinacea - The Immune Enhancer: Echinacea is perhaps one of the most well-known herbs for immune support. It's believed to increase the body's production of white blood cells, which fight infections.
    - o Echinacea Tea Recipe: Brew a tea using dried Echinacea flowers and leaves. Steep 1 teaspoon of the dried herb in hot water for about 10 minutes. Drinking this tea at the onset of cold symptoms can provide a boost to the immune system.

- Elderberry, The Antiviral Powerhouse: Elderberry is rich in antioxidants and vitamins and has been shown to combat viruses and shorten the duration of colds and flu.
    - o Elderberry Syrup Recipe: Simmer dried elderberries in water with a bit of cinnamon and ginger. After about 45 minutes, strain the mixture and add honey for sweetness. This syrup can be taken daily during flu season for preventive care.

- Astragalus, The Immune System Builder: Astragalus root is used in traditional Chinese medicine to strengthen the body against diseases. It's known for its ability to boost the immune system.
    - o Astragalus Root Decoction Recipe: Simmer sliced astragalus root in water for an hour. Strain and drink this decoction. It's best used as a preventative measure during the cold season.

Incorporating Immune-Boosting Herbs into Your Diet:

Apart from taking these herbs in tea or syrup form, there are other creative ways to include them in your diet.

- Herbal Smoothies: Add a teaspoon of elderberry syrup or Echinacea tincture to your morning smoothie. Blend it with fruits rich in Vitamin C to create an immune-boosting drink.

- Cooking with Herbs: Incorporate immune-supporting herbs like garlic, ginger, and turmeric into your cooking. These not only add flavor but also offer antimicrobial and immune-boosting properties.

- Herbal Soups and Broths: Make nourishing soups and broths with astragalus root, shiitake mushrooms, and other medicinal herbs. These can be particularly comforting and beneficial during the cold season.

Lifestyle Factors That Support Immunity:

In addition to herbal remedies, certain lifestyle practices can significantly boost your immune system.

- Balanced Diet: Ensure your diet is rich in fruits and vegetables, providing the necessary vitamins and minerals for a strong immune system.

- Regular Exercise: Moderate, regular exercise can enhance immune function and overall health.
- Adequate Sleep: Quality sleep is crucial for immune health. Aim for 7-9 hours of sleep per night.
- Stress Management: Chronic stress can weaken the immune system, making relaxation and stress-reduction practices essential.

In conclusion, this subchapter provides a thorough exploration of herbal remedies and lifestyle practices that can enhance your immune system, especially during the cold and flu season. By understanding and incorporating these natural solutions, you can proactively support your body's defense system. Remember, while these herbs and practices are beneficial for boosting immunity, they should be part of a comprehensive approach to health that includes regular medical check-ups and a healthy lifestyle.

SUMMER REMEDIES - HERBAL TREATMENTS FOR SEASONAL ISSUES.

Summer, with its warm weather and extended daylight hours, invites us outdoors but also brings along unique challenges like sunburn, insect bites, and heat-related issues. This subchapter focuses on herbal treatments tailored for these summer-specific concerns. By harnessing the power of natural herbs and ingredients, we can effectively and safely address these issues, making our summer experiences more enjoyable and comfortable.

Introduction to Summer Herbal Remedies:

The key to effective summer herbal remedies lies in understanding the properties of various herbs and how they can be applied to address common summer ailments. Herbs with cooling properties, natural antihistamine effects, and those that offer sun protection are particularly valuable during this season. Let's explore a range of herbal remedies, from soothing sunburns to repelling insects, each designed to enhance your summer health and wellness.

Herbal Remedies for Sunburn:

Sunburn can not only be painful but also damaging to the skin in the long term. Natural remedies can provide relief and aid in skin repair.

- Aloe Vera Gel for Immediate Relief: Aloe vera is renowned for its soothing and healing properties, making it an excellent remedy for sunburn.
    - Pure Aloe Vera Gel Application: Extract gel from an aloe vera leaf and apply it directly to the sunburned area. For a cooling effect, refrigerate the gel before application.

- Green Tea for Skin Repair: The antioxidants in green tea can help mitigate sun damage and soothe burned skin.
    - Green Tea Compress: Brew a strong pot of green tea and let it cool. Soak a clean cloth in

the tea and apply it as a compress to the sunburned areas.

- Calendula and Lavender Healing Salve: Both calendula and lavender have skin-healing and anti-inflammatory properties.
  - o Salve Recipe: Infuse calendula and lavender in a carrier oil like coconut or almond oil. Strain the herbs and mix the oil with beeswax to create a salve. Apply this to the sunburn to promote healing.

Herbal Treatments for Insect Bites and Stings:

Insect bites can be irritating and uncomfortable. Certain herbs can offer relief from itching and reduce inflammation.

- Basil Leaves for Itch Relief: Basil has compounds that provide relief from itching and swelling.
  - o Basil Leaf Poultice: Crush fresh basil leaves and apply them directly to the bite. Alternatively, make a tea with basil leaves, let it cool, and use it to rinse the affected area.

- Plantain for Natural Relief: Plantain, commonly found in yards and parks, is effective for insect bites and stings.
  - o Plantain Poultice: Crush fresh plantain leaves to release their juice and apply it to the bite or sting. This can quickly ease the itch and reduce swelling.

- Tea Tree Oil for Antiseptic Protection: Tea tree oil is a natural antiseptic and can help prevent bites from becoming infected.
  - Tea Tree Oil Application: Dilute tea tree oil with a carrier oil and apply it to the bite for relief and to prevent infection.

Herbal Remedies for Heat-Related Issues:

Staying cool and hydrated is essential during summer. Herbs can help in managing heat exhaustion and maintaining hydration.

- Peppermint Tea for Cooling: Peppermint has a natural cooling effect on the body.
  - Iced Peppermint Tea: Brew peppermint tea, let it cool, and serve it over ice for a refreshing and cooling summer drink.

- Cucumber and Mint Water for Hydration: Cucumbers and mint provide a hydrating and cooling effect.
  - Recipe: Add slices of cucumber and fresh mint leaves to water. Refrigerate and drink throughout the day to stay hydrated.

- Chrysanthemum Tea for Heat Relief: Chrysanthemum tea is known in traditional Chinese medicine for its cooling properties.

o   Brewing Chrysanthemum Tea: Steep dried chrysanthemum flowers in hot water, then cool and enjoy the tea to help lower body heat.

In conclusion, this subchapter provides an array of practical herbal remedies to combat common summer ailments such as sunburn, insect bites, and heat exhaustion. By integrating these natural solutions into your summer routine, you can address these issues safely and effectively, enhancing your enjoyment of the season. Remember, while these remedies are helpful for minor issues, severe reactions or persistent problems should be evaluated by a healthcare professional. Embrace these herbal strategies to make your summer experiences healthier and more enjoyable.

ADAPTING TO SEASONS - TAILORING HERBAL REMEDIES TO SEASONAL CHANGES.

In this subchapter we explore the concept of adapting herbal remedies and practices to align with the changing seasons. The natural world is in a constant state of flux, and our bodies are deeply connected to these seasonal cycles. By understanding how different seasons affect our health and wellbeing, we can utilize specific herbs and practices to maintain balance and harmony throughout the year.

Introduction to Seasonal Adaptation in Herbalism:

Seasonal adaptation in herbalism is about more than just addressing the typical health challenges of each season. It's about syncing our bodies with nature's rhythm. This alignment

155

can enhance our overall health, boost our immune system, and improve our emotional and physical resilience. Each season; spring, summer, autumn, and winter; brings its own energy and requires a different approach to health and wellness.

Spring: A Time of Renewal and Cleansing:

Spring is a time of awakening and renewal, both in nature and within our bodies. It's an ideal time for cleansing and rejuvenation after the winter months.

- Dandelion for Detoxification: Dandelion is a powerful detoxifier and is particularly beneficial for the liver.
  - Dandelion Tea Recipe: Steep the dried roots and leaves of dandelion in hot water. Drink this tea to help cleanse the body of toxins accumulated over winter.

- Nettle for Allergies: Spring often brings allergies. Nettle is a natural antihistamine and can help alleviate allergy symptoms.
  - Nettle Infusion: Soak dried nettle leaves in hot water overnight. Strain and drink this nutrient-rich infusion to combat seasonal allergies.

Summer: Focus on Cooling and Hydration:

Summer is characterized by warmth and increased outdoor activity, which can lead to issues like dehydration and overheating.

- Peppermint for Cooling: Peppermint is naturally cooling and can help the body regulate its temperature.
    - Iced Peppermint Tea: Brew peppermint tea, let it cool, and serve over ice. This refreshing drink is perfect for hot summer days.

- Cucumber Water for Hydration: Staying hydrated is crucial in the summer.
    - Cucumber Water: Add cucumber slices and mint to water. This not only flavors the water but also adds a cooling effect.

Autumn: Preparation for the Cold Months:

Autumn is a time to prepare the body for the colder months ahead. It's about nourishing and strengthening the body.

- Ginger for Immune Support: Ginger warms the body and boosts the immune system.
    - Ginger Tea with Honey: A simple ginger tea with a spoonful of honey can be both warming and immune-boosting.

- Turmeric for Inflammation: As the weather cools, inflammation can increase.

o   Golden Milk: Mix turmeric powder in warm
    milk with a pinch of black pepper. This drink is
    perfect for evenings and promotes overall well-
    being.

Winter: Immunity and Warmth:

Winter requires a focus on immune support and maintaining
warmth.

- Elderberry for Immune Boosting: Elderberry is
  excellent for preventing and treating colds and flu.
    o   Elderberry Syrup: Homemade elderberry syrup
        can be a delicious way to boost immunity
        during winter.

- Cinnamon and Clove for Warmth: These spices not
  only warm the body but also aid digestion.
    o   Spiced Herbal Tea: Add cinnamon and clove to
        your regular tea to create a warming,
        comforting beverage.

Adapting to the seasons with herbal remedies is a holistic
approach to health that aligns us with the natural cycles of our
environment. By understanding the specific needs of each
season and using herbs that are naturally available or
particularly effective during these times, we can optimize our
health year-round. This subchapter provides a comprehensive
guide to seasonal herbalism, offering practical and effective
ways to incorporate these natural solutions into your lifestyle.

Embrace these seasonal practices and herbs to live in greater harmony with the natural world and your own body.

Conclusion of the Book: Embracing a Journey of Herbal Healing and Wholeness

As we reach the conclusion, it is time to reflect on the journey we have embarked upon. This book has not only been a guide to the myriad herbal remedies and practices but also an invitation to embrace a lifestyle that is in harmony with nature and our own bodies. This conclusion aims to encourage readers to integrate the wisdom of herbal practices into their daily lives for long-term health and well-being, and to inspire continuous learning and exploration in the field of herbal medicine and holistic health.

The Path to Integrating Herbal Practices:

The journey towards holistic health is a personal and ongoing process. Integrating herbal practices into our daily lives is not about drastic changes but about making small, consistent shifts in how we approach our health and well-being. This can include:

- Incorporating Herbal Remedies: Start by incorporating simple herbal remedies into your routine. This could be a cup of herbal tea for relaxation, a herbal salve for skin care, or a natural remedy for a common ailment.

- Listening to Your Body: Pay attention to your body's responses to different herbs and treatments. Understanding your body's unique needs and reactions is key to effective herbal practice.

- Making Herbalism a Part of Daily Life: Herbalism isn't just about treating ailments; it's a way of life. This includes eating a balanced diet, engaging in regular physical activity, and adopting stress management techniques.

- Sustainable Practices: Be mindful of where and how you source your herbs. Opt for organic, ethically sourced herbs and consider growing your own.

Continuous Learning and Exploration:

The world of herbal medicine is vast and constantly evolving. Continuous learning and exploration are vital to deepening your understanding and practice.

- Educational Resources: Seek out books, courses, workshops, and online resources to expand your knowledge. Learning from different cultures and traditions can provide a broader perspective on herbal medicine.

- Community Engagement: Joining herbalism communities, whether local or online, can provide support, inspiration, and shared learning. Engaging with others on this path enriches the journey.

- Experimentation and Personalization: Herbal medicine is as much an art as it is a science. Feel encouraged to experiment with different herbs and formulations, always prioritizing safety and informed practice.

- Holistic Approach: Remember that herbal medicine is one part of a holistic approach to health. It works best in conjunction with other healthy lifestyle choices and, when necessary, conventional medical care.

Embracing a Life in Harmony with Nature:

Ultimately, embracing herbal practices is about more than just individual health; it's about living in a way that is in harmony with the natural world. It's a commitment to understanding and respecting the interconnectedness of our health with the health of our environment.

- Environmental Stewardship: As you grow in your herbal practice, consider how you can contribute to the health of the planet. This could be through sustainable gardening, supporting local herbalists, or advocating for environmental conservation.
- A Journey of Wholeness: Embracing herbalism is a journey towards wholeness, where health is viewed not just as the absence of disease but as a state of complete physical, mental, and social well-being.

In closing, this book is more than a book; it's an invitation to embark on a lifelong journey of discovery, healing, and harmony with the natural world. As you integrate these practices into your life, you join a community of individuals committed to a more natural, holistic way of living. May this journey bring you health, joy, and a deeper connection to the world around you.

EMBRACING HERBAL PRACTICES - INTEGRATING NATURE'S WISDOM FOR HEALTH AND WELL-BEING.

In this subchapter, we focus on the practical aspects of embracing herbal practices, guiding you to integrate these age-old traditions into your daily life for enhanced health and well-being. This journey isn't just about using herbs to treat ailments; it's about adopting a holistic lifestyle that connects you deeply with the healing power of nature.

Introduction to Integrating Herbal Practices:

Embracing herbal practices is more than just a choice; it's a transformational journey that aligns you with the rhythms of nature and your body. The art of herbalism is not only about understanding the properties of various herbs but also about learning how to incorporate them into your life seamlessly and effectively. This process involves a comprehensive approach, encompassing dietary changes, lifestyle adjustments, and a mindful connection with the environment.

Starting Your Herbal Journey:

- Understanding Herbal Properties: Begin by learning about different herbs and their properties. Books, online courses, and workshops can be invaluable resources. Focus on common herbs and their uses, gradually expanding your knowledge.

- Creating a Herbal Kitchen: Stock your kitchen with essential herbs. Start with versatile herbs like ginger, turmeric, garlic, and rosemary. These can be easily included in everyday cooking, offering both flavor and health benefits.

- Herbal Teas for Daily Health: Incorporate herbal teas into your daily routine. Chamomile for relaxation, peppermint for digestion, or green tea for antioxidants are excellent choices. Experiment with blends to find what works best for you.

Developing Herbal Routines:

- Morning Rituals: Start your day with a warm cup of lemon and honey water or a herbal tonic like ashwagandha or triphala. This can help cleanse your system and boost energy levels.

- Herbal Cooking: Use herbs in your cooking, not just for flavor but for their health properties. Include herbs like basil, thyme, and oregano in your meals. Experiment with different combinations to discover both the taste and health benefits.

- Evening Wind-Down: End your day with a calming herbal tea like lavender or valerian root, which can aid in relaxation and promote good sleep.

Incorporating Herbs into Self-Care:

- Herbal Baths: Add herbs like lavender or Epsom salts to your bath for relaxation and detoxification.

- Natural Skincare: Create simple herbal skincare products like calendula salve for skin healing or aloe vera gel for sunburn relief.

- Herbal Remedies for Common Ailments: Keep a small home herbal kit for common ailments. Include remedies like ginger tea for nausea, peppermint oil for headaches, and echinacea tincture for immune support.

Living in Harmony with Nature:

- Sustainable Herbalism: Practice sustainable herbalism by growing your own herbs or sourcing them from ethical, organic suppliers.

- Seasonal Herbalism: Adapt your herbal use according to the seasons. Use warming herbs like ginger in winter and cooling herbs like peppermint in summer.

- Connecting with Nature: Spend time in nature regularly. Gardening, hiking, or simply walking in a park can deepen your connection with the natural world.

Embracing herbal practices is a path to living a more balanced and harmonious life. It's about nurturing your body, mind, and spirit with the gifts of nature. As you integrate these practices into your daily routine, you'll discover a deeper sense of well-being and a renewed connection to the world around you. Remember, this journey is personal and evolving. Be patient and open to learning and experiencing new aspects of herbalism as you go along. Here's to your health, happiness, and the rewarding journey ahead in the world of herbal healing.

Continuous Learning and Exploration - A Lifelong Journey in Herbal Medicine and Holistic Health

Embarking on a journey in herbal medicine and holistic health is not just a one-time endeavor, but a lifelong process of learning, exploration, and personal growth. This subchapter is dedicated to inspiring and guiding you to continuously expand your knowledge and understanding of herbal medicine and holistic health practices. It's about fostering a sense of curiosity and a desire for ongoing education, ensuring that your journey in herbalism is ever-evolving and deeply enriching.

Introduction to Lifelong Learning in Herbalism:

The field of herbal medicine is vast and rich with history, knowledge, and continuous advancements. Whether you are a beginner or have been practicing herbalism for years, there is always something new to learn and explore. This commitment to ongoing education is crucial not only for personal growth but also for the safe and effective use of herbal medicine.

Establishing a Foundation for Continuous Learning:

- Building a Herbal Library: Start by creating a personal library of herbal books, journals, and resources. Include classic herbal texts as well as contemporary studies and articles.

- Joining Herbal Communities: Become part of herbalist communities, both online and in person. Forums, social media groups, and local herbal clubs can provide support, inspiration, and shared knowledge.

- Attending Workshops and Seminars: Regularly attend workshops, seminars, and conferences on herbal medicine and holistic health. These events are great opportunities to learn from experienced practitioners and to network with peers.

Deepening Herbal Knowledge and Practice:

- Exploring Herbal Traditions: Study various herbal traditions from around the world such as Traditional Chinese Medicine, Ayurveda, Western herbalism, and Native American herbal practices. Each tradition offers unique perspectives and remedies.

- Cultivating a Medicinal Herb Garden: If space allows, grow your own medicinal herb garden. This hands-on experience is invaluable for understanding plant growth, harvesting, and the properties of herbs.

- Experimenting with Herbal Preparations: Practice making your own herbal preparations such as tinctures, salves, teas, and infusions. Document your recipes and their effects for future reference.

Integrating Holistic Health Practices:

- Combining Herbs with Nutrition: Learn about the interplay between herbal medicine and nutrition. Explore how dietary choices can complement herbal remedies and vice versa.

- Incorporating Mind-Body Practices: Experiment with integrating mind-body practices like yoga, meditation, or Tai Chi into your routine. These practices can enhance the effectiveness of herbal treatments.

- Understanding Modern Medicine: Stay informed about how herbal medicine intersects with conventional medical practices. This knowledge is essential for ensuring safety, especially when dealing with chronic conditions or when combining herbal remedies with other medications.

Staying Informed and Safe:

- Keeping Up with Research: Regularly read scientific studies and research papers on herbal medicine. This will help you stay updated on the latest findings and safety information.

- Engaging with Herbal Experts: Seek mentorship or guidance from experienced herbalists. Their insights and experiences can be invaluable in your learning journey.

- Educating Others: Share your knowledge with others. Teaching can be a powerful way to deepen your understanding and appreciation for herbal medicine.

As you continue on this path of discovery in herbal medicine and holistic health, remember that every step forward is an opportunity to deepen your connection with nature and with your own body. The journey of learning in herbalism is infinite, filled with wonders, insights, and transformations. Embrace this path with an open heart and mind, and let your passion for herbal medicine and holistic health guide you to a fulfilling and enlightened existence. Your journey is not just about personal healing, but also about contributing to a healthier, more balanced world.

LAST WORDS: A CONGRATULATORY NOTE AND WORDS OF ENCOURAGEMENT.

As we turn the final pages of this book, it is both a moment to reflect and to celebrate. You, the reader, have embarked on a remarkable journey through the pages of this book, exploring the profound wisdom of herbal healing and holistic practices. Congratulations on completing this journey! This accomplishment speaks volumes about your dedication to personal health, well-being, and a deeper connection with the healing powers of nature.

A Testament to Your Commitment:

By reaching this point, you have shown a commendable commitment to enhancing your health and that of those around you. Whether you are new to herbalism or have been exploring it for some time, your journey through this book has equipped you with valuable knowledge and practical skills that can significantly impact your life and the lives of others.

The Book as a Lifelong Companion:

Remember, this book is not just a one-time read. It's a companion for life, a treasure trove of wisdom that you can return to time and again. The recipes, remedies, and insights

171

provided here are meant to be revisited, each time deepening your understanding and practice of herbal medicine.

Implementing Recipes at Your Pace:

Start implementing these recipes and practices at a pace that feels comfortable for you. Even if you begin by incorporating just a few of these remedies into your routine, you are taking significant steps toward a healthier lifestyle. Every small change, every single herb used, every moment spent connecting with the natural world contributes to your journey towards wellness and harmony.

Awareness and Influence:

By embracing the teachings of this book, you are not only improving your own life but also becoming a beacon of awareness and health in your community. Remember, many people are still unaware of the powerful benefits of herbal healing. Your knowledge and experience, no matter how small you may think it is, can inspire and educate others.

Looking Forward with Hope and Wisdom:

As you move forward, carry the wisdom from this book in your heart. Let it guide you in your daily life, influence your decisions, and shape your journey towards health and happiness. You are now part of a community that values health.

respects nature, and believes in the power of herbal medicine to transform lives.

Final Words of Encouragement:

In closing, we extend our heartfelt congratulations and encourage you to continue your journey with enthusiasm and curiosity. Keep exploring, keep learning, and keep implementing these practices. Your journey through this book is just the beginning. Here's to your health, your growth, and your continued journey in the wonderful world of herbal healing and holistic well-being.

Important information! Why Our Book Does Not Include colored Herb Photos!

Consideration for Cost and Accessibility:

In our commitment to keeping the book affordable, we consciously decided against including color herb photos. This decision directly impacts and lowers the printing costs, making the book more accessible to a broader range of readers. Our priority is to provide comprehensive herbal knowledge at a reasonable price.

Emphasizing the Role of Visual Aids:

Understanding the importance of visual identification in herbal studies, especially for newcomers and in recipe preparation, we recommend for detailed herb images.

https://myplantin.com/plant-identifier/herb

This online resource complements our book perfectly, enabling accurate herb identification and enhancing your herbal learning experience.

Appendices: A Treasure Trove of Herbal Knowledge.

As we conclude, the Appendices serve as a valuable resource, a final chapter that complements and enhances the rich content of this book. This section is designed to be a practical and accessible reference, assisting you in your ongoing journey with herbal medicine and natural healing. It encapsulates the essence of the book, offering concise and essential information that can be referred back to time and time again.

The Appendices are crafted with the intention of providing ease and clarity in your herbal practice. Whether you are a seasoned herbalist or a newcomer to this fascinating world, you will find these resources to be an invaluable addition to your herbal library. The information here is organized to support quick retrieval and easy understanding, making your experience with herbal remedies both enjoyable and effective.

In these Appendices, you will discover a compilation of tools and references that encapsulate the wisdom of the entire book. It's a section that brings together the practical aspects of herbal medicine, offering a quick yet comprehensive guide to the vast array of herbal recipes discussed throughout the book. This section ensures that the knowledge you've gained is always within reach, ready to assist you in your daily practices and explorations.

Furthermore, the Appendices provide a quick reference guide to the most commonly used herbs, detailing their properties, uses, and benefits. This guide is a handy tool for both beginners and experienced practitioners, offering a quick way to recall the specific qualities and applications of each herb. It's an essential resource that will enhance your understanding and utilization of herbal medicine.

Lastly, for those who wish to delve deeper and broaden their knowledge, the Appendices include a curated list of further learning resources. This list encompasses books, websites, and other materials that have been carefully selected to enrich your journey in herbal wisdom and natural healing. These resources are a gateway to further exploration, offering diverse perspectives and deeper insights into the art and science of herbalism.

In essence, the Appendices of this book are not just an addition but an integral part of your journey with herbal medicine. They are here to guide, assist, and inspire you as you continue to explore the enriching path of natural healing and wellness.

HERBAL RECIPE GUIDE, A COMPREHENSIVE COMPILATION.

Welcome to the first section of our Herbal Recipe Guide, an integral part of the Appendices. This guide serves as a comprehensive directory to all the herbal recipes included in our book, meticulously organized from A to Z for your convenience. This segment provides easy access to a wealth of herbal knowledge, ensuring that the power of natural healing is always at your fingertips.

A: Herbal Recipes Starting with 'A'

- Aloe Vera Gel for Skin Healing: Extract the gel from an aloe vera leaf and apply it directly to soothe burns, cuts, or skin irritations.

- Ashwagandha Tonic for Stress Relief: Mix half a teaspoon of ashwagandha powder in warm milk or water. Drink before bedtime to help reduce stress and improve sleep quality.

- Apple Cider Vinegar Tonic for Digestion: Mix two tablespoons of apple cider vinegar in a glass of water. Drink before meals to aid digestion.

- Arnica Salve for Bruises and Sprains: Infuse arnica flowers in a carrier oil, strain, and mix with beeswax to create a salve. Apply to bruises and sprains to reduce swelling and pain.

B: Herbal Recipes Starting with 'B'

- Basil Tea for Headache Relief: Steep fresh or dried basil leaves in boiling water. Drink the tea to alleviate headache symptoms.

- Burdock Root Decoction for Detoxification: Simmer burdock root in water for 30 minutes. Drink this tea to help detoxify the liver and improve skin health.

- Bilberry Extract for Eye Health: Use bilberry extract as per the recommended dosage for improving eye health and vision.

- Black Cohosh Tea for Menopause Relief: Brew black cohosh in hot water to make a tea. Drink to alleviate menopause symptoms like hot flashes and mood swings.

C: Herbal Recipes Starting with 'C'

- Chamomile Tea for Relaxation: Infuse chamomile flowers in hot water. Drink before bed to promote relaxation and improve sleep quality.

- Calendula Cream for Skin Care: Infuse calendula petals in a carrier oil, blend with beeswax and shea butter to create a soothing skin cream.

- Cinnamon Infusion for Blood Sugar Control: Steep cinnamon sticks in boiling water. Drink daily to help regulate blood sugar levels.

- Clove Oil for Toothache Relief: Dilute clove oil with a carrier oil and apply to the affected tooth for temporary relief from toothache.

D: Herbal Recipes Starting with 'D'

- Dandelion Tea for Liver Support: Brew dried dandelion root and leaves to make a detoxifying tea. It supports liver function and digestion.

- Devil's Claw Tincture for Arthritis: Use devil's claw tincture as directed to help alleviate joint pain and symptoms of arthritis.

E: Herbal Recipes Starting with 'E'

- Echinacea Tincture for Immune Boosting: Take echinacea tincture as per guidelines to enhance immune system function, especially during cold and flu season.

- Elderberry Syrup for Cold and Flu: Simmer dried elderberries with water and honey to make a syrup. Take during the cold and flu season for prevention and treatment.

F: Herbal Recipes Starting with 'F'

- Feverfew Tea for Migraine Relief: Steep dried feverfew leaves to make a tea. Drink to prevent or alleviate migraine headaches.

- Fennel Seed Tea for Digestive Health: Infuse fennel seeds in hot water to make a tea that aids digestion and relieves bloating.

- Flaxseed Poultice for Skin Inflammation: Mix ground flaxseeds with water to form a paste. Apply as a poultice to inflamed or irritated skin areas.

G: Herbal Recipes Starting with 'G'

- Ginger Tea for Nausea Relief: Simmer slices of fresh ginger in water for 15 minutes. Strain and add honey for a soothing tea that relieves nausea and aids digestion.

- Garlic Infusion for Immune Support: Steep minced garlic in hot water for a potent drink that boosts the immune system and combats colds.

- Ginkgo Biloba Extract for Cognitive Health: Consume ginkgo biloba extract as per recommended dosage to enhance memory and cognitive function.

- Goldenseal Tincture for Digestive Issues: Use goldenseal tincture to alleviate digestive problems, but adhere to the recommended dosages due to its potent nature.

H: Herbal Recipes Starting with 'H'

- Hawthorn Berry Tea for Heart Health: Brew hawthorn berries to create a heart-supportive tea, known for improving cardiovascular function.

- Horsetail Decoction for Bone Health: Simmer horsetail in water to make a tea that supports bone and joint health due to its high silica content.

- Holy Basil (Tulsi) for Stress Reduction: Brew holy basil leaves to create a stress-relieving and balancing herbal tea.

- Hibiscus Tea for Blood Pressure Management: Regularly drink hibiscus tea to help manage blood pressure levels and for its high antioxidant content.

I: Herbal Recipes Starting with 'I'

- Ivy Leaf Cough Syrup for Respiratory Health: Boil ivy leaves and mix with honey to create a syrup that relieves cough and supports respiratory health.

J: Herbal Recipes Starting with 'J'

- Juniper Berry Tea for Urinary Tract Health: Infuse juniper berries in hot water to make a tea that supports urinary tract health and has diuretic properties.

K: Herbal Recipes Starting with 'K'

- Kava Kava Beverage for Anxiety Relief: Prepare a kava kava beverage by steeping its root. It's known for its calming effects but should be consumed responsibly due to its potent nature.

- Kratom Tea for Pain Relief: Use kratom leaves to brew a tea for pain relief. Note: Kratom's legal status varies by region and it should be used with caution.

L: Herbal Recipes Starting with 'L'

- Lavender Infusion for Relaxation: Steep lavender flowers in hot water to make a calming tea, ideal for reducing stress and promoting relaxation.

- Lemon Balm Tea for Digestive Comfort: Brew lemon balm leaves for a soothing tea that aids digestion and relieves symptoms of indigestion.

- Licorice Root Tea for Sore Throat Relief: Make a tea with licorice root, which is effective in soothing sore throats and coughs.

- Linden Flower Tea for Relaxation and Sleep: Infuse linden flowers in boiling water to create a tea that helps with relaxation and promotes restful sleep.

M: Herbal Recipes Starting with 'M'

- Mint Tea for Digestive Relief: Brew fresh or dried mint leaves for a refreshing tea that soothes digestive discomfort and eases nausea.

- Milk Thistle Extract for Liver Health: Regularly use milk thistle extract, as directed, to support liver health and detoxification.

- Marshmallow Root Infusion for Respiratory Support: Steep marshmallow root in hot water to create a soothing mucilage beneficial for coughs and sore throats.

- Motherwort Tincture for Heart Health: Consume motherwort tincture, following recommended dosages, to support heart health and reduce anxiety.

N: Herbal Recipes Starting with 'N'

- Nettle Leaf Tea for Allergy Relief: Infuse dried nettle leaves to make a tea that naturally combats allergic reactions and boosts overall immunity.

- Neem Oil for Skin Health: Apply diluted neem oil to the skin to combat acne and skin infections due to its antibacterial properties.

O: Herbal Recipes Starting with 'O'

- Oregano Oil for Immune Support: Use oregano oil diluted in a carrier oil as a potent antibacterial and antiviral remedy, especially effective during cold and flu season.

- Oat Straw Infusion for Nervous System Support: Steep oat straw in hot water to create a nourishing drink that supports nerve health and reduces anxiety.

P: Herbal Recipes Starting with 'P'

- Peppermint Oil for Headache Relief: Apply diluted peppermint oil to temples and forehead for natural relief from tension headaches.

184

- Passionflower Tea for Insomnia: Brew dried passionflower to make a calming tea, ideal for promoting restful sleep and reducing anxiety.

- Pau d'Arco Tea for Antifungal Support: Make a tea from Pau d'Arco bark to leverage its antifungal and immune-boosting properties.

- Plantain Poultice for Skin Healing: Crush fresh plantain leaves and apply as a poultice to soothe insect bites, cuts, and skin irritations.

Q: Herbal Recipes Starting with 'Q'

- Quassia Bark Digestive Tonic: Simmer quassia bark to create a tonic that stimulates digestion and combats intestinal parasites.

R: Herbal Recipes Starting with 'R'

- Rosehip Tea for Vitamin C Boost: Brew dried rosehips for a tea rich in Vitamin C, ideal for immune support and skin health.

- Raspberry Leaf Tea for Women's Health: Steep red raspberry leaves to make a tea that supports female reproductive health and eases menstrual discomfort.

- Rhodiola Extract for Stress Reduction: Take rhodiola extract as directed to help combat fatigue and reduce the effects of stress on the body.

- Rosemary Hair Rinse for Scalp Health: Infuse rosemary in water and use as a final hair rinse to stimulate hair growth and improve scalp health.

S: Herbal Recipes Starting with 'S'

- St. John's Wort Tincture for Mood Support: Use St. John's Wort tincture, as directed, to help alleviate mild to moderate depression and uplift mood.

- Sage Tea for Throat Health: Brew dried sage leaves for a tea that offers antiseptic properties, ideal for sore throats and oral health.

- Slippery Elm Bark for Digestive Soothing: Prepare a soothing drink with slippery elm bark powder to ease digestive discomfort and acid reflux.

- Saw Palmetto Extract for Prostate Health: Consume saw palmetto extract as per recommended guidelines to support prostate health.

T: Herbal Recipes Starting with 'T'

- Thyme Infusion for Respiratory Health: Steep thyme leaves in hot water for a tea that helps clear respiratory passages and fight coughs.

- Turmeric Milk for Anti-Inflammatory Benefits: Mix turmeric powder in warm milk with a pinch of black pepper for a drink that combats inflammation and boosts overall health.

- Tea Tree Oil Application for Skin Infections: Dilute tea tree oil with a carrier oil and apply to skin areas affected by fungal infections or acne.

U: Herbal Recipes Starting with 'U'

- Uva Ursi Tea for Urinary Tract Support: Brew uva ursi leaves to create a tea beneficial for urinary tract infections and kidney health.

V: Herbal Recipes Starting with 'V'

- Valerian Root Tea for Sleep Aid: Infuse valerian root in hot water to make a tea that promotes relaxation and aids in treating insomnia.

- Vervain Tincture for Nervous System Support: Use vervain tincture, as directed, to help relieve stress and calm the nervous system.

W: Herbal Recipes Starting with 'W'

- Witch Hazel Compress for Skin Healing: Apply witch hazel extract to a cloth and use as a compress for skin irritations, hemorrhoids, and varicose veins.

- White Willow Bark Tea for Pain Relief: Steep white willow bark to create a tea that acts as a natural pain reliever, similar to aspirin.

- Wild Yam Cream for Hormonal Balance: Apply wild yam cream topically as directed to help balance hormones and ease menopausal symptoms.

- Wormwood Tincture for Digestive Health: Consume wormwood tincture in small doses to stimulate appetite and improve digestion.

X: Herbal Recipes Starting with 'X'

- Xanthoparmelia Scabrosa Extract: Used in traditional medicine, this extract is often taken as directed for specific health conditions. It's important to use under professional guidance due to its potent nature.

Y: Herbal Recipes Starting with 'Y'

- Yarrow Tea for Fever and Cold: Brew yarrow flowers and leaves to make a tea that is effective in reducing fever and aiding in cold and flu symptoms.

- Yellow Dock Root Tonic for Anemia: Simmer yellow dock root to create a tonic that is beneficial for its iron content and can help in cases of mild anemia.

- Ylang-Ylang Oil for Stress Relief: Use ylang-ylang essential oil in aromatherapy or dilute with a carrier oil for topical application to help reduce stress and anxiety.

- Yohimbe Bark Extract for Circulatory Health: Yohimbe bark extract is sometimes used to improve circulation, but it should be used cautiously and under the guidance of a healthcare professional due to its potent effects.

Z: Herbal Recipes Starting with 'Z'

- Zedoary Root Tea for Digestion: Brew zedoary root, a relative of turmeric, to make a tea that aids digestion and relieves flatulence.

- Zinc-Rich Herbal Blend for Immune Support: Combine herbs high in zinc such as pumpkin seeds, echinacea, and garlic to create a blend that supports the immune system.

- Ziziphus Jujuba (Jujube) for Sleep: Consume jujube fruit or tea before bedtime to help improve sleep quality due to its calming properties.

- Zingiber Officinale (Ginger) for Nausea: Ginger, in various forms such as tea, capsules, or fresh root, is effective in treating nausea and digestive issues.

Each of these recipes offers a glimpse into the vast and versatile world of herbal medicine. They are intended to be both practical and easily integrated into daily life, providing natural solutions for a range of health concerns. Whether you're looking to improve sleep, support digestion, or maintain skin health, these recipes can be a valuable part of your wellness toolkit. As you explore and utilize these herbal remedies, remember to consider your unique health needs and consult with a healthcare professional when necessary.

As you reach the end of this guide, consider it a beginning rather than a conclusion. The world of herbal remedies is expansive and ever-evolving, with each herb offering its own unique properties and health benefits. This guide serves not just as a resource but as a source of motivation for you to continue your exploration into the healing powers of nature. It's an invitation to discover and implement new methods to enhance your health and well-being using the wisdom of herbal medicine.

HERBAL INGREDIENTS QUICK REFERENCE, A COMPREHENSIVE GUIDE.

This part of the appendices in is dedicated to a quick reference guide for the most commonly used herbs and their properties. Spanning from A to Z, this guide offers an extensive list of herbs, each with its unique qualities and uses in herbal medicine. This compilation serves as a practical tool for quick reference and a deeper understanding of the myriad herbs at your disposal.

A: Common Herbs and Their Properties

- Aloe Vera: Known for its soothing, healing properties, particularly for skin issues like burns and cuts.
- Ashwagandha: An adaptogen, supports stress relief and improves energy levels.
- Astragalus: Boosts the immune system and has anti-inflammatory properties.
- Arnica: Used topically for bruises, sprains, and muscle soreness.
- Angelica: Known for digestive health benefits and used in treating colds.
- Anise: Beneficial for digestion and respiratory health.

B: Common Herbs and Their Properties

- Basil: Antioxidant-rich, aids in digestion and can alleviate stress.

- Burdock Root: Detoxifies the blood and promotes skin health.
- Black Cohosh: Used for women's health issues, particularly menopause symptoms.
- Bilberry: Supports eye health and circulation.
- Borage: Contains anti-inflammatory properties and supports adrenal health.

C: Common Herbs and Their Properties

- Chamomile: Calming, aids in sleep, and helps with digestive issues.
- Calendula: Anti-inflammatory, used for skin healing and soothing.
- Cayenne: Stimulates circulation and aids in pain relief.
- Cinnamon: Balances blood sugar levels and has antimicrobial properties.
- Comfrey: Known for skin healing and supporting bone health.

D: Common Herbs and Their Properties

- Dandelion: Supports liver health, detoxification, and is a natural diuretic.
- Devil's Claw: Used for pain relief, particularly in joints and muscles.
- Damiana: Known as a mood enhancer and aphrodisiac.
- Dong Quai: Often used in women's health for menstrual and menopausal issues.

E: Common Herbs and Their Properties

- Echinacea: Enhances the immune system and fights infections.
- Elderberry: Antiviral, commonly used for colds and flu.
- Eyebright: Traditionally used for eye irritations and maintaining good vision.
- Eucalyptus: Beneficial for respiratory health, used in decongestants.

F: Common Herbs and Their Properties

- Fennel: Aids in digestion and is effective against bloating and gas.
- Feverfew: Used for migraine relief and reducing fever.
- Flaxseed: High in omega-3 fatty acids, beneficial for heart and digestive health.
- Frankincense: Anti-inflammatory, used in skin care and for calming the mind.

G: Common Herbs and Their Properties

- Ginger: Renowned for its digestive benefits, anti-inflammatory properties, and effectiveness in nausea relief.
- Ginkgo Biloba: Known for improving cognitive function and circulation.
- Garlic: Offers immune-boosting properties and is beneficial for cardiovascular health.

- Ginseng: Used for energy enhancement and stress reduction.
- Goldenseal: Contains antibacterial properties, often used for digestive and respiratory issues.

H: Common Herbs and Their Properties

- Hawthorn: Supports heart health and is used for cardiovascular conditions.
- Horsetail: Rich in silica, beneficial for bone, hair, and nail health.
- Holy Basil (Tulsi): An adaptogen, helps in stress relief and enhances overall vitality.
- Hibiscus: Used for blood pressure management and is rich in antioxidants.
- Hyssop: Beneficial for respiratory health, often used in cough remedies.

I: Common Herbs and Their Properties

- Ivy Leaf: Used in respiratory health, especially in treating coughs and bronchitis.
- Irish Moss: Known for its high mineral content, beneficial for thyroid health and as a source of natural collagen.

J: Common Herbs and Their Properties

- Juniper Berry: Diuretic properties, used for urinary tract health and detoxification.
- Jasmine: Often used in aromatherapy for its calming properties and in skin care.

K: Common Herbs and Their Properties

- Kava Kava: Known for its sedative properties, used to reduce anxiety and promote relaxation.
- Krishna Tulsi: Similar to Holy Basil, used for its adaptogenic and stress-relieving properties.
- Kudzu: Used in traditional medicine for alcoholism treatment and for its anti-inflammatory effects.

L: Common Herbs and Their Properties

- Lavender: Widely known for its calming and relaxing properties, beneficial for anxiety, sleep, and skin health.
- Lemon Balm: Offers calming effects, assists in digestion and is often used to relieve stress.
- Licorice Root: Beneficial for digestive health and adrenal support.
- Linden Flower: Often used for calming nerves, reducing anxiety, and aiding sleep.

M: Common Herbs and Their Properties

- Mint: Known for its digestive benefits and soothing properties, especially for stomach discomfort and irritable bowel syndrome.
- Milk Thistle: Prominent for liver health, it aids in detoxification and liver cell regeneration.
- Marshmallow Root: Soothes mucous membranes, beneficial for respiratory and digestive tract irritation.
- Mullein: Often used in respiratory health for its expectorant properties, aiding in coughs and bronchial congestion.
- Motherwort: Known for its use in heart health and menstrual discomfort relief.

N: Common Herbs and Their Properties

- Nettle: Rich in nutrients, it's beneficial for allergies, hair health, and as a general tonic.
- Neem: Widely used for its antibacterial and antifungal properties, particularly in skin care.
- Nutmeg: Used in small quantities for digestive health, but should be used cautiously due to its potent effects.
- Noni: Known for its immune-boosting and anti-inflammatory properties.

O: Common Herbs and Their Properties

- Oregano: Contains potent antimicrobial properties, often used in respiratory and digestive health.
- Olive Leaf: Known for its cardiovascular benefits and as a natural antiviral and antibacterial agent.

- Oat Straw: Nourishing for the nervous system, it's used for stress relief and to enhance mood.

P: Common Herbs and Their Properties

- Peppermint: Widely used for digestive issues, including IBS, nausea, and indigestion.
- Parsley: Rich in vitamins, beneficial for kidney health and as a natural diuretic.
- Plantain: Used topically for skin irritations and bites, and internally for digestive health.
- Passionflower: Known for its calming effects, useful for anxiety and sleep disorders.

Q: Common Herbs and Their Properties

- Quassia: Used for digestive health, particularly for stimulating appetite and aiding digestion.
- Quince: Traditionally used in treating gastrointestinal disorders and as an anti-inflammatory agent.

R: Common Herbs and Their Properties

- Rosehip: High in Vitamin C, used for immune support and skin health.
- Raspberry Leaf: Known for women's health, particularly during pregnancy and for menstrual discomfort.

- Rhodiola: An adaptogen, used for stress relief, energy enhancement, and mental focus.
- Rosemary: Enhances memory and concentration, also used for its anti-inflammatory and antioxidant properties.

S: Common Herbs and Their Properties

- Sage: Known for its antioxidant properties, sage is beneficial for cognitive health and digestion.
- St. John's Wort: Commonly used for its mood-lifting properties, particularly in mild to moderate depression.
- Saw Palmetto: Often used for men's health, particularly for prostate health and balancing hormone levels.
- Slippery Elm: Soothes the digestive tract and is helpful in cases of acid reflux and gastrointestinal inflammation.
- Spearmint: Similar to peppermint, it aids in digestion and is milder, suitable for sensitive individuals.

T: Common Herbs and Their Properties

- Thyme: Has strong antimicrobial properties, often used for respiratory infections and coughs.
- Turmeric: Known for its potent anti-inflammatory properties and beneficial in various health conditions, from arthritis to digestive issues.
- Tansy: Traditionally used as a worm expellant and for menstrual issues, but should be used cautiously.

U: Common Herbs and Their Properties

- Uva Ursi: Often used for urinary tract health, particularly in cases of infections due to its antiseptic properties.
- Usnea: Known for its antimicrobial properties, particularly used in respiratory and skin infections.

V: Common Herbs and Their Properties

- Valerian Root: Widely recognized for its sedative qualities, valerian is often used in sleep aids and for anxiety relief.
- Verbena: Known for its calming effects, helpful in reducing stress and aiding digestion.
- Violet: Used both internally and externally, it is beneficial for respiratory health and skin conditions.

W: Common Herbs and Their Properties

- Witch Hazel: Widely used as a topical astringent for skin issues, including acne and inflammation.
- White Willow Bark: Known as a natural pain reliever, it contains salicin, which is similar to aspirin.
- Wild Yam: Often used in women's health for its potential to balance hormones and relieve menopausal symptoms.
- Wood Betony: Traditionally used for headaches and nervous system support.

X: Common Herbs and Their Properties

- Xanthoparmelia Scabrosa: Often used in traditional remedies, it's known for various therapeutic properties. However, it is less common and should be used under professional guidance.

Y: Common Herbs and Their Properties

- Yarrow: A versatile herb used for its wound-healing properties, it also aids in fever reduction and improves digestion.
- Yellow Dock: Known for its benefit to skin health and as a blood purifier, it's also used to improve digestion and liver function.
- Yucca: Traditionally used for its anti-inflammatory properties, particularly in joint and skin health.
- Yerba Mate: A popular herb for its energizing properties, it's also rich in antioxidants and nutrients.

Z: Common Herbs and Their Properties

- Zedoary: A lesser-known relative of turmeric, used for its anti-inflammatory and digestive properties.
- Ziziphus (Jujube): Valued for its calming properties and used to improve sleep quality and reduce anxiety.
- Zingiber (Ginger): Widely known for its digestive benefits, anti-inflammatory properties, and effectiveness against nausea.

- Zea Mays (Corn Silk): Traditionally used for urinary tract health and as a mild diuretic.

This guide is designed to be a quick yet comprehensive reference to the world of herbs, aiding you in identifying the right herb for your health needs. Each entry provides a snapshot of the key properties and uses of these common herbs, making it an invaluable resource for anyone interested in herbal medicine. As you familiarize yourself with these herbs, you'll find them to be essential allies in your pursuit of wellness and harmony.

FURTHER LEARNING RESOURCES

As you reach this juncture, it's clear that the journey into herbal wisdom and natural healing is an ever-evolving path. This final subchapter is dedicated to providing you with a curated list of further learning resources. These resources are selected to deepen your understanding and expand your knowledge in the realms of herbal medicine and holistic health.

Books and Publications by Barbara O'Neill:

- "Self Heal By Design" by Barbara O'Neill: This book offers insights into how the body can heal itself naturally and delves into various aspects of natural health and lifestyle changes that can facilitate this process.

- "The Ultimate Health Program" by Barbara O'Neill: Here, O'Neill provides comprehensive guidance on nutrition, exercise, herbal remedies, and other natural health strategies.

Recommended Books on Herbal Medicine and Natural Healing:

- "The Way of Herbs" by Michael Tierra: This book is an excellent resource for understanding herbal medicine, covering both theory and practical applications.

- "Medical Herbalism: The Science and Practice of Herbal Medicine" by David Hoffmann: A comprehensive guide that blends the scientific aspects with traditional knowledge in herbal medicine.

- "Encyclopedia of Herbal Medicine" by Andrew Chevallier: An extensive resource detailing the use of 550 herbs and remedies for common ailments.

Lectures and Talks:

- Barbara O'Neill's Health and Wellness Seminars: Available online, these seminars cover a wide range of topics from detoxification to mental health, emphasizing the role of diet and natural remedies.

- Webinars and Online Courses: Various platforms offer webinars and courses on herbal medicine, where experts share their knowledge and latest research findings.

Online Resources and Websites:

- HerbMentor: An online community for herbal learning which offers courses, videos, and articles.

- Mountain Rose Herbs Blog: A comprehensive resource for herbal recipes, wellness tips, and herbal lore.

- The Herbal Academy: Offers online herbalism programs ranging from introductory to advanced levels.

Podcasts and YouTube Channels:

- "Herbal Radio" by Mountain Rose Herbs: A podcast dedicated to the world of herbs and herbalism.

- "The Plant Path" by The School of Evolutionary Herbalism: A podcast that dives deep into the world of herbal medicine and holistic healing.

By exploring these resources, you can continue to expand your knowledge and understanding of herbal medicine and holistic health practices. Each book, course, and lecture offers a unique perspective, empowering you with the tools and wisdom to further your journey in natural health and wellness. Remember, the path of learning is infinite, and each step you take enriches your journey in the beautiful world of herbal wisdom.

The End.
Margaret Willowbrook.

A MESSAGE FROM THE PUBLISHER:

Are you enjoying the book? We would love to hear your thoughts!

Many readers do not know how hard reviews are to come by and how much they help a publisher. We would be incredibly grateful if you could take just a few seconds to write a brief review on Amazon, even if it's just a few sentences!

Please go here to leave a quick review:

https://amazon.com/review/create-review?&asin=B0CT8R6KHQ

We would greatly appreciate it if you could take the time to post your review of the book and share your thoughts with the community. If you have enjoyed the book, please let us know what you loved the most about it and if you would recommend it to others. Your feedback is valuable to us, and it helps us to improve our services and continue to offer high-quality literature to our readers.

Made in the USA
Las Vegas, NV
02 March 2024

86605110R00125